Treatment of the ever-increasing variety of addic
a wide range of psychotherapeutic and cognitive-behaviou
Over recent years, initiatives have been established critica **14 DAY**
the usefulness of psychotherapy in many areas of psychia\ **BOOK**
serves as a timely review of psychological treatments in t
and provides a rare combination of expertise both from a\
cialists and those in other fields who use psychotherapeutic approaches to
treat a broad variety of personal problems. Its coverage includes contextual ideas that are basic to any approach to therapy, and an exploration
of particular treatment strategies. Throughout, this volume is able to
provide both authoritative statements and to engage the reader in the
excitement of debate. It forms a valuable reference that is sure to appeal
to a wide range of practitioners and researchers concerned with alcohol
and drug problems as well as to therapists in other areas.

PSYCHOTHERAPY, PSYCHOLOGICAL
TREATMENTS AND THE ADDICTIONS

PSYCHOTHERAPY, PSYCHOLOGICAL TREATMENTS AND THE ADDICTIONS

Edited by

GRIFFITH EDWARDS

National Addiction Centre
Institute of Psychiatry, University of London

and

CHRISTOPHER DARE

Section of Psychotherapy, Institute of Psychiatry,
University of London

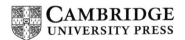

CAMBRIDGE
UNIVERSITY PRESS

Published by the Press Syndicate of the University of Cambridge
The Pitt Building, Trumpington Street, Cambridge CB2 1RP
40 West 20th Street, New York, NY 10011-4211, USA
10 Stamford Road, Oakleigh, Melbourne 3166, Australia

First Published 1996

Printed in Great Britain at the University Press, Cambridge

A catalogue record for this book is available from the British Library

Library of Congress cataloguing in publication data

Psychotherapy, psychological treatments, and the addictions / edited
by Griffith Edwards and Christopher Dare.
p. cm.
Includes index.
ISBN 0 521 55357 1 ((hardcover). – ISBN 0 521 55675 9 (pbk.)
1. Substance abuse – Treatment. 2. Psychotherapy. I. Edwards,
Griffith. II. Dare, Christopher.
[DNLM: 1. Psychotherapy – methods. 2. Behavior, Addictive –
therapy. 3. Substance Abuse – therapy. 4. Alcoholism – therapy.
WM 420 P9758245 1996]
RC564.P87 1996
616.86'0651 dc20
DNLM/DLC
for Library of Congress 95–23014 CIP

ISBN 0 521 55357 1 hardback
ISBN 0 521 55675 9 paperback

KW

Contents

Contents

Contributors

K. Eia Asen
Maudsley Hospital, Denmark Hill, London SE5 8AZ, UK

Christopher Dare
Section of Psychotherapy, Institute of Psychiatry, De Cespigny Park, London SE5 8AF, UK
(and Maudsley and Bethlem NHS Trust, Denmark Hill, London SE5 8AZ)

Robin Davidson
Holywell Hospital, 60 Steeple Road, Antrim BT41 2RJ, Northern Ireland

Susan Davison
Maudsley and Bethlem NHS Trust, Denmark Hill, London SE5 8AZ, UK

Griffith Edwards
National Addiction Centre, Addiction Sciences Building, 4 Windsor Walk, London SE5 8AF, UK

Wojciech Falkowski
St George's Hospital and Medical School, Jenner Wing, Cranmer Terrace, London SW17 0RE, UK

Gill Gorell Barnes
Tavistock Centre, 120 Belsize Lane, London NW3 5BA, UK

Michael Gossop
National Addiction Centre, Addiction Sciences Building, 4 Windsor Walk, London SE5 8AF, UK

Kingsley Norton
Henderson Hospital, 2 Homeland Drive, Sutton, Surrey, UK (and St George's Hospital Medical School, Jenner Wing, Cranmer Terrace, London SW17 0RE, UK)

Harvey Ratner
Brief Therapy Practice, 4d Shirland Mews, Maida Vale, London W9 3DY, UK

Julian Stern
Department of Psychotherapy, Maudsley Hospital, Denmark Hill, London SE5 8AF, UK

Stephen Sutton
Health Behaviour Unit and National Addiction Centre, Addiction Sciences Building, 4 Windsor Walk, London SE5 8AF, UK

Ruth Williams
Department of Psychology, Institute of Psychiatry, De Crespigny Park, London SE5 8AF, UK

Dennis Yandoli
Unit 5, 1/31 Elkstone Road, London W10 5NT, UK

George E. Vaillant
Division of Psychiatry, Brigham and Women's Hospital, 75 Francis Street, Boston, Massachusetts 02115, USA

Psychotherapy and psychological treatments of substance problems: generalism, specialism and the building of bridges

The need for bridges

The purpose of this book is to assist in the building of bridges between two important sectors of psychotherapeutic endeavour. One of these comprises the vastly wide background of activity that deals with the generality of intra- and interpersonal problems and discomforts. Our second area of concern is the specialised psychotherapeutic work that aims at helping individuals and families who are encountering difficulties with alcohol or other drugs.

The degree of separation that exists between the substance problems and generalist worlds of practice will vary across time and country, and within any one country there will be variations at the local level. Whatever the particular circumstances, the situation that pertains is likely to represent some variant on the relationship between off-shore island and the mainland. In some instances there may be ample bridges and free movement between the two areas. On other occasions the picture seems more to suggest that the bridges have fallen down with the inhabitants of the island isolated, evolving their own narrow culture, and neither visiting nor visited by the dwellers on the mainland.

To characterise the situation as universally one where no communication exists would be nihilistic to the point of absurdity. Forces, however, exist that may often be more favourable to the building of barriers than to the construction of bridges between groups of workers for whom mutual communication potentially offers great advantage.

One influence towards separation derives from the fact that in many countries the system that delivers care for patients with drug or alcohol problems is physically separate from the facilities that deal with the generality of psychotherapeutic work. The specialist and generalist practitioners will not often meet at lunch-time. Moreover, the separation is not just at the level of any single day's work or contact, but is cumulative and a matter of career.

The loss that can result from the decay of communications is likely to effect both sides of the divide. Alcohol and other drug workers have skills and rich experience that can profitably be shared with the wider treatment community. In complimentary fashion the specialist substance practitioners should be seeking a continued updating in their awareness of generic developments, while also looking for insights that may come from contact with other specialist groups such as colleagues working with eating disorders, with delinquent or acting-out young people, or with clients who are suffering from the sequelae of sexual abuse.

Psychotherapy and psychological treatment: merging another divide

In the general field the term 'psychotherapy' is probably most commonly used to describe forms of treatment that acknowledge the importance of working with transference relationships. The meaning of the term has changed in the face of a loosening of orthodoxies and broadening of practice content, so that strict definition becomes more difficult. The term 'behaviour therapy' might at first sight appear to be more self-evidently definable. It started out as a set of approaches that took the individual's behaviour as the target problem. What went on within the black box of the psyche was excluded from consideration. The distinction between psychotherapy and behaviour therapy as drawn in those terms is absolute. However, with the emergence of cognitive behavioural approaches, many ways of working are being developed that make productive connections across what was always a somewhat spurious divide. If besides its prime purpose of assisting the bridging between substance misuse and the generalist mainland we have a secondary purpose or a sub-plot, it will be to break down unhelpful barriers between psychotherapy and psychological treatments.

How this book came about, and its structure

This book derives from a one-week seminar held at the National Addiction Centre, London. The presentations were planned to support the purposes that now come through as those of this book. Some new material has been added.

A proportion of the chapters focus on generic issues and others on substance problems. We have purposely mixed together the two kinds of presentations, believing that in this mixing and merging lies the play. Sometimes chapters rather easily provide a generalist/specialist pairing, but in other instances it did not seem helpful to set things up this way. We believe that the job of exploring the relevance of what the generalists say for the professional activities of the substance specialists (and vice versa), lies best with the individual reader and we have not interrupted the text with passages that impose any set of editorial interpretations. Like the meeting from which this book derives, the intention is to invite an active and personal involvement in reflection, debate, and weighing of evidence.

The structure of the book is as follows. Part one is headed 'Backgrounds to Therapeutic Understanding'. While holding off from detailed consideration of practice and techniques, this group of presentations explores contextual ideas that will bear on how we approach therapy, whatever the specifics.

Part two, **Treatments**, deals with an array of general and specialist treatment approaches including psychotherapy as traditionally defined, cognitive-behaviour therapy, family and couples work, group therapy, the processes of Alcoholics Anonymous, motivational issues and the phasing of treatment, and how therapeutic communities work.

Part three offers a postscript under the title A small group experience. We hope this contribution will help to give further reality to our intention of a debate that actively involves its readership. The background meeting started each day with scheduled small group discussions. This final chapter is an account of what happened in one such group.

Acknowledgements

We are grateful to the 36 participants from several different countries who participated in the London seminar. Their input valuably contributed to the shaping of this book. The organisation of that meeting was managed by Seta Durguerian. Secretarial assistance in the preparation of this text has been handled by Patricia Davis. We are grateful to Jocelyn Foster who has been our link with Cambridge University Press. Financial assistance for this project was generously and exclusively provided by Roche Pharmaceuticals.

Part one

Backgrounds to therapeutic understanding

1

Addictions over the life course: therapeutic implications

GEORGE E. VAILLANT

Introduction

Previous longitudinal studies (O'Donnnell, 1969; Maddox and Desmond, 1981; Vaillant, 1983; Edwards, 1984; Fillmore, 1988) have considered how alcohol and heroin abuse began, the factors that maintained these addictions, and how recovery is eventually achieved. Previous publications, but quite different ones, have addressed the issue of adult development (e.g. Vaillant, 1977, 1993). Indeed, over the past 25 years the monographs addressing adult development are far too many to cite.

What is missing, however, is a consideration of the relationship between adult development and substance abuse. In addressing this relationship and its therapeutic implications one must be tentative. Reliance must be placed on inadequate, parochial and sometimes speculative data. Often, even when the conclusions are empirically grounded, they will depend on data from a 50-year follow-up (Vaillant, 1983, 1995) of two relatively small cohorts of American men. Nevertheless, the relationship between substance abuse and adult development is important enough to examine with the data available. Only if and when the pioneering studies of adolescent drug use and abuse by Richard Jessor (1987) and Denise Kandel (1985) have survived for 50 years will we have an empirical basis with which really to address the questions posed in this chapter.

The greatest obstacle to understanding the relationship between adult development and the paths out of drug abuse is the impact of secular changes upon drug use. In many ways drug abuse is more like fashion – a result of historical whim – than a result of biology and thus susceptible to development forces. For example, it would be hard to tie women's choice of footwear to adult development. In the 1940s, young women wore plimsoles (the ancestors of running shoes) and the very old wore 'granny' boots. In the 1990s, the very old wear running shoes and

3

young women wear 'granny' boots. In analogous fashion, in the late 1950s in Japan, there were up to 60 000 arrests a year for methamphetamine misuse; in the 1960s, when methamphetamine abuse was no longer in fashion, arrests for methamphetamine abuse sank to 200. By 1985, the number of methamphetamine arrests in Japan have again increased to 20 000 (Miller and Kozel, 1991). In other words, both onset and offset of methamphetamine abuse in Japan had more to do with the effects of historical fashion than with adult development or with therapy.

In the United States the seemingly lawful effects of social class upon cigarette abuse in young adults have changed within a generation. In the 1940s, among college students, cigarette use was highest among those from upper-middle-class family backgrounds (McArthur *et al.*, 1958) and less common among young adults from blue-collar backgrounds. In advertisements, middle-aged doctors seemed plausible when they asserted that Camels were good for their 'T-zone' (larynx). Currently, the same upper-middle-class birth cohort, especially the doctors, have largely given up smoking; whereas middle-aged blue-collar males continue to smoke heavily. Medical and social fashions, not adult maturation, have been the instrument of change.

Having thus warned the reader that all the generalisations in this chapter about the relationships of adult development to drug abuse are vulnerable to error, variables will be identified that do tie adult development to drug use and recovery.

In this chapter it is argued that the life course of adult drug abuse is analogous to a polydrug abuser's use of multiple agents during the course of a single day. Stimulants are used to wake up in the morning, cigarettes and alcohol are consumed socially at lunch and sedatives are used to calm down at the end of the day. Put more directly, in the morning of life adolescent drug abusers use drugs for their capacity to produce novelty, excitement, and to open new avenues of experience. In middle life, drug abuse is more purely social and more closely linked to social ritual. In late life, drug use is used to produce quiet, preserve sameness and to reduce the implications of novelty and change (Pascarelli, 1981). As a reflection of this hypothesized pattern the ratio of drug abuse to alcohol abuse as a reason for admission to American Veteran's hospitals declines from 1:2 before age 35 to 1:25 between 55 and 65 and then, admission due to abuse of prescription drugs goes down to 1:20 after 65 (Moos *et al.*, 1993). In Japan, inhalant abuse peaks before age 20, methamphetamine abuse before 35, hypnotic abuse at age 40 and antianxiety drugs at age 55

(Fukui *et al.*, 1988). The highest use of hypnotic, pain-relieving and tranquillizing medications occurs in men and women after age 60 (Blazer, 1989). However, *illicit* drug abuse is almost non-existent for those over 60 (Robins and Regier, 1991).

Onset of abuse

In early adolescence, the first drugs of abuse are inhalants, e.g. glue. These agents simply produce a rapid change in state. Their use is quickly followed by psychedelics and stimulants that produce novel experiences, and drugs like crack cocaine and heroin that are not only associated with excitement but also with deviant, and hence novel lifestyles. In the United States over the last 30 years, the sequence of inhalant abuse, to marijuana and alcohol abuse, to cocaine abuse has remained constant. The mean age of onset of abuse of each of the four agents has remained the same. (O'Donnell *et al.*, 1976; Gfroer and Brodsky, 1992).

Second, licit drug *use* usually precedes illicit drug *use*, but illicit drug *abuse* may precede licit drug *abuse*. Although much of the criminal activity seen in alcoholics is a product of alcohol abuse (Vaillant, 1983), heroin abusers are antisocial prior to onset of drug abuse (Vaillant, 1966). In the United States in 1910 heroin abuse, before it was illegal, was just as firmly linked to youthful crime as it is today (Lichtenstein, 1914). As a general rule of thumb, if illicit drug use has not taken place before age 25, it will not occur (Kandel, 1978). This same generalisation holds true for larceny, for car theft and initiation into motorcycle gangs. The earlier criminal behaviour begins, the earlier illicit drug use will begin and the later into the life cycle both behaviours will continue.

In marked contrast, almost all the commonly abused drugs of old age – sedative drugs, tranquillizers and hypnotics – are obtained legally and through socially accepted channels. In men especially, the use of licit psychoactive drugs increases in linear fashion until age 75 (Josephson and Caroll, 1974).

As a result, the treatment of drug abuse in the young depends upon diverting illicit behaviour into acceptable paths and providing non-pharmacological alternatives for the adolescents' need to dissociate and produce change of state for its own sake. In the United States, group activities like the Red Berets (adolescents who police underground trains) and Outward Bound have been effective in combating adolescent drug abuse on a small scale. However, such adolescent needs can only be permanently met by the self-efficacy and environmental control that comes with maturity. The most common alternative is for adolescent drug experimentation to be replaced with interpersonal intimacy. Such a process is epitomised by the drinking song: 'Wedding bells are breaking up that old gang of mine'.

To relieve drug abuse in old age, the therapeutic challenges are quite different. Novelty and danger need to be reduced not enhanced. Dependency needs become more salient and adolescent counter-dependency needs become almost non-existent.

Initiation of drug abuse over the life course

Having made these generalisations, there are four variables that must be considered in order to understand the relationship of adult development to shifting patterns of drug abuse. The first variable is an increasing tolerance for depression over the life course. The second variable is the decline in antisocial behaviour over the adult life course. The third variable is the increasing capacity for intimacy that occurs during adult development. The fourth variable is the power that schedules of reinforcement exert over drug effects.

These variables must be addressed one at a time. First, the ability to tolerate and to hold sad feelings in consciousness, and the ability to manifest depressed affect in honest and not self-destructive or disguised ways, increases progressively over adult life. Expressed in terms of normal development, adolescents often deal with depression, loss, and dysphoria by seeking a change in state. This may be achieved by intoxication, excitement, and defensive anger towards others. Whereas, in mid-life, thanks to life experience and to brain muturation, individuals are more able to tolerate the fact that their dysphoria lies within themselves. Instead of externalising pain, they internalise it. In accepting responsibility for their depression they may initially turn their defensive anger against themselves but later they may merely seek honest relief from their own despair. Thus, as young adults mature there is a shift from drugs that provide distraction from depression to those that provide solace. Such individuals evolve from seeking illicit drugs to change state, to seeking prescription drugs to relieve depression, to developing mature relationships and self-soothing activities like religion in order to bear grief through non-pharmacological means.

Before adolescence, both boys and girls from very disrupted family envionments are likely to manifest conduct disorder. By adolescence, women from such environments tend to become self-destructive and are often diagnosed as masochistic or depressed. In contrast, adolescent males continue to manifest antisocial externalising behaviours. After age 40, many former male delinquents experience clinical depressions. In late life, both sexes often can tolerate the sorrow of their youth without self-medication.

As a result of such factors, illicit drug abuse is most common among antisocial male adolescents; abuse of licit drugs is most common among depressed young women from abusive or disrupted families. Indeed, primary alcohol abuse is often misdiagnosed major depressive disorder – especially in women. After age 30, both depression and abuse of licit drugs (alcohol and tranquillizers), continues to be common among the previously antisocial from both sexes. With maturity, socially acceptable clinical depression takes the place of histrionic tantrums. Alcohol, that once was used as a stimulant and thus stimulus for adolescent escapism, in the middle years, used as a sedative, only makes suicidal rumination and anhedonia worse. This change in the experienced effects of self-medication with alcohol may facilitate hitting bottom.

The increasing salience of depressive symptomatology over the adult life course can be appreciated in the natural history of the psychiatric symptomatology of progressive, genetically determined brain diseases like Huntington's chorea. When penetrance of the single, dominant, autosomal gene of Huntington's chorea occurs in adolescence, the first psychiatric symptoms are most often antisocial behaviour. When the first penetrance of the gene occurs in the 20s the symptoms often reflect a schizophreniform psychosis. After age 30, the first psychiatric effects of the gene's penetrance are often manifested as major depressive disorder (Weinberger, 1987).

Second, and related to the first point, antisocial behaviour declines over the adult life course. Thus, over time, maturity allows illicit drugs to be replaced by licit drugs. Both environmental and biological factors affect such development. On the one hand, what we call sociopathy, or social deviance, or Bohemianism, is more often seen among the socially neglected, the socially dislocated, and the socially disadvantaged, but such behaviour is also more often seen among adolescents in heart if not in years. Social deviance and violation of adult convention is less usual before age 12 and after age 40. Social deviance probably peaks between the years of 14 and 18 and is highly correlated with illicit drug use. The personality traits that Cloninger refers to as being low on harm-avoidance and high on novelty-seeking (Cloninger, 1987) probably peak at these same ages. At 60, characteristically, the same individuals are more likely to be high in harm-avoidance and low in novelty-seeking, and, of course, they are less likely to use illicit drugs.

To generalise, the more antisocial *or* socially deviant *or* familially abused the individual, the greater the variety of drugs he or she will have used before age 25, the earlier such drugs will have been used, the more likely they are to be abused. The reason for this strong relationship of deviance to polydrug abuse can be conceptualised within the sociological model as due to anomie, social deviance, violating public canons, and seeking novel forms of excitement. Or it can be explained within the medical, sick-role model as due to seeking relief from environmental and intrapsychic conflict and from clinical depression. The greater the individual's pain, the more widely will they use and abuse available pharmacological agents. Thus, the severely abused child evolves into polydrug abuse whether as a teenage prostitute or Borstal boy. Twenty years later, the same indviduals are likely to be help-rejecting complainers eliciting polypharmacy from their general physician.

In part, social deviance is a reflection of the use of excitement and dissociation by young adults as an antidepressant. Change of state is achieved most effectively by rapid- and short-acting drugs. Such drugs hasten dependence. For example, heroin *use* occurs after the *use* of most other drugs, including alcohol, yet heroin *dependence* occurs at a mean age of about 20, whereas the mean age of alcohol *dependence* and severe nicotine dependence occurs perhaps a decade later. Thus, deviance can dramatically shorten the time between use and abuse.

Licit and illicit abuse of the same drug can peak at different ages. Among alcohol abusers *per se*, although *abuse* occurs much earlier among sociopaths than among college graduates, *use* occurs at almost the same age (Vaillant, 1994). The mean age for the onset of illegal opiate abuse (usually heroin) is 20, whereas the mean age of the 'legal' opiate abuse (in the USA usually Demerol), which is seen most often now in physicians and still seen in iatrogenic addicts, occurs at age 35–40.

Indvidual recreational drug choice will change with the fashions, but only the established polydrug *abuser* will go on to use the most rapid-acting and self-injurious agents. While the sequence to be described below was applicable for American males during the 1970s (O'Donnell *et al.*, 1976), and the percentages are only approximate, the principles may be generalisable. Fifty per cent of alcohol users have *never* used other recreational drugs including marijuana. Ninety percent of marijuana users, however, have used alcohol, but 50% have *never* used other recreational drugs (i.e. sedatives, stimulants, and hallucinogens). Ninety per cent of individuals using hallucinogens, stimulants, and sedatives, have used marijuana, but 50% have never used cocaine. Ninety per cent of cocaine users, have used or abused the major recreational drugs, but 50% have *never* used heroin or crack cocaine. Ninety per cent of heroin *users* have *abused several* other major classes of recreational drugs.

Third, maturity allows 'masturbatory' drug use to be replaced by real relationships. Among the young, drug use and abuse may take the place of, or ward off, intimate relationships. Most often drug use of this sort occurs in a social context. On the one hand, drugs are often used in the service of the developmental task of overcoming the anxieties associated with social encounter with non-family members. In young men, drunkenness and incipient alcohol abuse is often 'cured' by marriage. Adolescent substance abuse can sometimes be abandoned on falling in love. On the other hand, drug use after the age of 45 is often a solitary activity, and has more to do with the pain of being with oneself rather than with others. Joint pain, failed life dreams and insomnia, are far greater burdens to a 65-year-old than is what to say to the neighbours at the general store or on the front porch. In contrast, adolescents put up with motorcycle injuries and insomnia without great anxiety and still believe that their dreams will come true, while they may find social encounters in high-school corridors and dating bars excruciating.

Fourth, the effect that a given drug has on an individual is very much dependent on the behaviour and setting of the individual. For example, legal amphetamines produce tranquillity among hyperactive children in a classroom; the same drugs obtained illegally produce over-stimulation in college students in social settings. To relieve dysphoria the young may abuse 'sedative' drugs to produce excitement, change of state, and to turn anger outwards; in middle-life 'sedative' drugs are used more directly for their hypnotic and numbing qualities. Alcohol is a stimulant when imbibed with others at a soccer match or in a bar room; alcohol is a sedative if imbibed alone in front of the television set. Among the old, barbiturates are used as hypnotics; among the young, barbiturates are used to 'party'.

Maintenance of drug abuse during the life course

To understand the course of drug addiction, it is important to study community samples, rather than clinical samples. The reason for this is that clinical samples are always severely biased. First they are more likely to include addicts comorbid for other disorders. Second, clinic cohorts are more likely to over-sample the chronically relapsing addict. Third, addicts who have achieved abstinence no longer come to clinics. Thus, clinic samples are more likely to focus attention on treatment failures and the mentally ill rather than on natural healing processes among the psychiatrically average.

From a one- or two-year perspective, established drug dependence in a clinic population appears to be a chronic, non-remitting process. Clinic interventions do not last, and in some studies of heroin addiction relapse is as high as 97%. What is striking, however, about substance dependence in community samples over the life course is its instability (Maddox and Desmond, 1981; Fillmore, 1987). When looked at over 20 years or more of follow-up, one study suggested that only about one alcohol- or heroin-dependent person in five is still actively using (Vaillant, 1988). This finding was in spite of the fact that only socially disadvantaged inner-city samples were studied. The instability of drug dependence over the long-term results from the fact that usually severe dependence leads to abstinence or death.

However, recent findings (Vaillant, 1995) suggest that alcohol *abuse* in middle life, in contrast to *dependence*, may be relatively chronic. A cohort of socio-economically favoured men was selected in college for mental health and followed for a lifetime. Although they often began abusing alcohol in middle-life, a majority continued abusing alcohol until death. Of the 10 out of 52 men who achieved stable abstinence, all had been alcohol dependent (DSM-III criteria). In contrast, socially disadvantaged inner-city alcoholics, many of whom appeared sociopathic, become addicted younger and were more likely to become dependent; but they were twice as likely to develop stable abstinence as the more advantaged college sample.

Recovery from addiction during the life course

There is no specific age at which drug or alcohol abusers recover. The notion that addicts 'burn out' in middle life is a misinterpretation of relatively smooth attrition among drug-dependent individuals. Such attrition comes both from a doubled rate of death and from the roughly 2% of addicted individuals who make a stable recovery each year. Cigarette abusers provide the clearest illustration. Neither maturation nor formal treatment has much effect upon nicotine dependence, but compared to 20–30-year-olds, relatively few 70–80-year-olds smoke two packs of cigarettes a day (Gomberg, 1990). The reason is both accelerated mortality and the fact that heavy smokers eventually discover techniques to maintain stable abstinence.

As is the case with smoking cessation, the critical factors in abstinence from other addictions do not seem to be maturation, treatment, or even a stable premorbid personality or social adjustment. Rather, recovery seems to depend both upon the severity of the addiction and upon the individual either encountering the right kind of naturalistic healing experience, or premature death. In one longitudinal study (Vaillant, 1994), by age 60 or 70 only about 20% of the nicotine-dependent men were still smoking and only 20% of the alcohol-abusing men were still abusing alcohol. These parochial findings are supported by the fact that only about 1% of addicts in methadone programmes are over age 60, and in a national sample of Americans only about 6% of alcoholics were over 60 (Robins and Regier, 1991). One reason for this decline, of course, is the inexorable mortality that is associated with substance abuse, but it is also due to stable abstinence. However, long-term follow-up of both heroin abusers and alcohol abusers reveals that there are very few predictors that distinguish the stably abstinent from the chronic addict.

Let's first eliminate four factors that play at best only a minor role in long-term outcome. First, people do not grow out of alcohol abuse or heroin abuse any more than they grow out of nicotine abuse or obesity or any other firmly entrenched habit. Studies of middle-aged men over one to two decades do not reveal diminution of mean alcohol consumption over time (Blazer, 1989). Second, addicts do not give up substance abuse because they 'burn out'. It is true that at the end of the life cycle, severe illness can lead to abstinence from cigarettes, alcohol, and heroin; but that is not how most addicts recover. Third, people do not recover because of a favourable past. In short-term studies, premorbid social stability is a powerful predictor of the response to treatment. However, such favourable response does not always last. In their long-term follow-up of heroin addicts, Maddox and Desmond (1981) found that premorbid factors did not distinguish those who became stably abstinent and those who did not. In a study of 150 alcoholics followed until late middle life, neither premorbid risk factors for alcoholism, nor premorbid factors like social stability, predicted outcome at age 60 (Vaillant, 1994). Fourth, stable recoveries from drug dependence are only sometimes the result of formal treatment interventions. If this seems astonishing, consider our limited success in treating obesity and nicotine dependence.

Rather, there seem to be three very disparate general factors that contribute to stable remission; but these factors can operate at any stage in
the life cycle. The first factor is experiencing very mild drug abuse; the
second is experiencing very severe dependence. Both conditions are statistically associated with good outcomes – but for very different reasons
(Edwards *et al.*, 1988). It is probably the combination of these two factors
that cancel out the effect of premorbid social stability on outcome. The
third factor consists of a cluster of life experiences described below, that
minimise relapse.

Let's look at these three factors one at a time. First, if drug abuse is
mild and of short duration, a simple change in life circumstances may
lead to complete remission. If early on in a drug-using career, before
habits are entrenched, one's social environment dramatically changes –
e.g. return from Vietnam (Robins, 1974), or abandoning a motorcycle
gang for a marital dyad – stable remission can occur.

Second, if drug abuse is very severe, stable abstinence becomes more
likely. It is paradoxical that severity (i.e. 'getting tired of getting sick and
tired', or 'hitting bottom') should be a favourable factor. But two-pack-a-
day smokers are at least as likely to give up smoking as one-pack-a-day
smokers and probably more likely to give up smoking than true social
smokers or those who use pipes and cigars. In following 25 late-onset
socially privileged alcohol abusers without dependence for 50 years and
16 early-onset sociopathic alcohol-*dependent* men for a similar length of
time, none of the former and 50% of the latter became abstinent or
returned to controlled drinking (Vaillant, 1995). However, perhaps the
latter had more reason to stop. Edwards and colleagues (1988) have
noted the same phenomenon.

The third factor is the fortuitous occurrence in the addict's life of four
life experiences that disrupt entrenched habits. These experiences include
acquiring a substitute behaviour that competes with the addiction,
encountering compulsory supervision or an 'external super ego', discovering new and most often religious sources of hope and self-esteem, and
finding new people to love to whom the addict is not 'in debt'. These four
experiences are found most reliably in cognitive behavioural treatment
programmes and in Alcoholics Anonymous (AA). In their literature
reviews of remission from abuse of tobacco, food, opiates, cocaine and
alcohol, Brownell *et al.* (1986), Stall and Biernacki (1986) and Miller
(1993) all identify these four life experiences as important.

Each of these naturalistic healing experiences needs to be described in
greater detail. The first experience is finding a reinforcing behaviour that

competes with drug use (e.g. meditation, compulsive gambling, overeating, etc.). It is no accident that the coffee-drinking, cigarette-smoking and self-esteem-building AA meetings are scheduled to occur during peak drinking hours. Second, being offered compulsory supervision or experiencing a consistent behavioural modification programme (e.g. use of disulfiram or a painful ulcer or a cognitive-behavioural relapse prevention programme) seems valuable (Miller, 1993). This is because although willpower is important in seeking treatment and for brief cessation of drug use, willpower is *not* associated with successful relapse prevention. Successful relapse prevention, like liberty, depends upon eternal vigilance. Thus, relapse prevention is best achieved by obtaining external reminders (e.g. parole, support groups or behaviour modification). For example, a first step in smoking cessation is to tell all your friends you are stopping – to make your decision public. Third, inspirational group membership (e.g. discovering a sustained source of hope, inspiration and self-esteem in fundamentalist religion or AA), seems important to maintaining behaviour change and stable reaction formations. (By reaction formation is meant the cognitive and affective reversal that occurs when a once-pleasurable instinctual goal (e.g. cigarette smoking) becomes disgusting.)

Fourth, during recovery it is valuable for addicts to form bonds with people they have not hurt in the past. The formation of a new stable relationship with a non-blood relative is often associated with stable abstinence. In this regard an AA sponsor, a support group or a new spouse may be more useful than the dyadic relationship with a long-suffering family member, which must repeatedly reawaken old guilts and old angers – conditioned reinforcers of alcohol use. Thus, marital couples therapy is not particularly useful in facilitating abstinence from alcoholism (Orford and Edwards, 1977; Vaillant, 1983).

The same four experiences were found among lives of the abstinent heroin addicts in Maddox's long-term study (Maddox and Desmond, 1981). Of those heroin addicts stably abstinent, 42% had a year of parole (compulsory supervision); 43% of those stably abstinent had used alcohol as a *substitute* for heroin and many others were in methadone maintenance programmes; 17% of the stably abstinent were working to treat other addicts in agencies (i.e. finding people for whom to care for whom they were not in 'debt'), and 25% became involved in evangelical religious activities. *Each* of those four circumstances also occurred in about 50% of the abstinent heroin and alcohol addicts in other long-term follow-up studies (Vaillant, 1968, 1988).

As already suggested, these four mutually reinforcing circumstances are also found in AA and in similar self-help organisations. Indeed, it is noteworthy that in an eight-year follow-up study by William Miller, a former critic of AA, of 140 patients trained to return to controlled drinking, only 10% did so successfully; however, 16% became successfully abstinent. Of the 13 of his 140 patients who subsequently made 100 visits to AA, 54% were among those who became stably abstinent ($p < 0.01$) (Miller *et al.*, 1992).

Finally, there is the paradoxical fact that therapeutic intervention in drug abuse may be more successful at age 35 than at 60. Youthful substance abusers by reason of immaturity and their use of rapid-acting drugs are less in control, and thus more subject to the ego dystonic effects of the drug. Thus, although stable abstinence may not occur for 10 or 20 years, abstinence is more frequent in those who began abuse when young. In contrast, the legal, somewhat comforting, substance abuse engaged in by the middle-aged, is much harder to treat and it has a worse prognosis, perhaps because it is more ego syntonic. Consider the analogy of suicidal behaviour. The unhappy, socially deviant young person is frequently suicidal in ways that require societal intervention; society insists upon suturing up self-inflicted wrist slashes and requiring motorcycle helmets. But the very painful, self-destructive qualities of such adolescent behaviours allow the individual to hit bottom, which leads to their eventual extinction. The blatantly self-detrimental behaviour associated with severe substance dependence allows us to intervene with some confidence. The 20-year-old rescued from the window ledge of a skyscraper thanks us. He had wished to change his state, not to die.

In contrast, the 85-year-old seeking suicide – from his Hemlock Society, or her Dr Kevorkian – would regard our interference a violation of civil rights. Sigmund Freud, when young, took cocaine to feel strong and alive; when, after a decade, he recognised cocaine was foe and not friend, he stopped. Sigmund Freud, when old and in pain, instructed his physician, Max Schur, to administer an overdose of morphine. It was an ego syntonic decision, and I am sure that Freud viewed the morphine as a friend not foe.

Thus, drug abuse in the elderly may sometimes become a part of what they have to live for, rather than a reflection of what they are trying to live against. They may wish to smoke themselves to death; and while their misuse of sedatives and alcohol remains distressing to their relatives, it remains a comfort to themselves. In short, the misuse of drugs by the elderly is *relatively* controlled and *relatively* a function of mature experience. Thus, interventions must be undertaken with empathy and with attention as to what the individual truly wishes. At the same time, doctors need to use special care in prescribing psychoactive drugs in the elderly (Blazer, 1989). *Much of the licit drug abuse by the elderly is iatrogenic and not a result of personal choice – especially in nursing homes.*

Conclusions

In summary, there are several trends that can be observed in drug use and abuse over the life course. First, over time there is a gradual shift from using drugs to excite the self and to change state, to using drugs to sedate the self and to preserve the status quo. Second, inhalants, both glue and cigarette smoking, are the first drugs of abuse to be used. The mean age of onset of most of the stimulant drugs occurs before age 20, while the peak use of sedative drugs in the population occurs after age 45 (Pascarelli, 1981). Third, although legal drug *use*, if not legal drug *abuse*, almost always precedes illegal drugs use, the more antisocial the individual the earlier illegal drug abuse will begin. Fourth, the young, by adjusting their behavioural repertoire, use alcohol and barbiturates as excitatory, rather than as sedative, drugs. Fifth, due to their use of rapid-acting agents to change state, drug use is more likely to evolve into dependence among the young than among the old. Sixth, the cessation of drug abuse depends in part upon the maturing individual being able to bear depression and to replace 'masturbatory' self-soothing drug ingestion with intimate relationships. Seventh, cessation of drug dependence often requires major changes in life circumstances. Individuals do not simply mature out of severe drug dependence. Granted, that the greater tolerance of depression and of intimacy that comes with maturity will help; but addicted individuals often also require external supervision *and* substitute dependencies *and* increased religious involvement *and* new love relationships too.

Would-be therapists of substance abusers must learn to work with these natural sources of recovery. AA and similar organisations that encompass these four factors must be regarded as powerful allies not competitors. As the last word, perhaps a study by Mann *et al.* (1991) will be illuminating. In a multivariate comparison of the declining cirrhosis rates in contrasting American states, they noted that such declines were independently correlated with increases in AA membership and with decreases in alcohol consumption but not with increased rates of utilisation of professional treatment services. As Orford and Edwards (1977) suggest when treating the addictions, we need to work with naturalistic healing forces, not in competition with them.

Acknowledgement

This work was supported by research grants KO5-MH00364 and MH42248 from the National Institute of Mental Health.

Bibliography

Blazer, D. G. (1989) Alcohol and drug problems in the elderly. In: Busse, E.W. and Blazer, D. G. (eds.) *Geriatric Psychiatry*, pp. 489–511. Washington DC: American Psychiatric Press.

Brownell, K. D., Marlatt, G. A., Lichtenstein, E. and Wilson, G. T. (1986) Understanding and preventing relapse. *American Psychologist*, **41**, 765–82.

Cloninger, C. R. (1987) Neurogenetic adaptive mechanisms in alcoholism. *Science*, **236**, 410–16.

Edwards, G. (1984) Drinking in longitudinal perspective: career and natural history. *British Journal of Addiction*, **79**, 175–83.

Edwards, G., Brown, D., Oppenheimer, E., Sheehan, M., Taylor, C. and Duckitt, E. (1988) Long-term outcome for patients with drinking problems: the search for predictors. *British Journal of Addiction*, **83**, 917–27.

Fillmore, K. M. (1987) Women's drinking across adult life course as compared to men's: a longitudinal and cohort analysis. *British Journal of Addiction*, **83**, 801–12.

Fillmore, K. M. (1988) *Alcohol Use Across the Life Course*. Toronto: Addiction Research Foundation.

Fukui, S., Watanabe, N., Iyo, M. *et al.* (1988) An epidemiological survey of drug dependence. In: *1987 Report of Studies of Etiological Factors and Pathological Conditions of Drug Dependence*, pp. 169–82. Tokyo: Ministry of Health and Welfare.

Gfroer, J. and Brodsky, M. (1992) The incidence of illicit drug use in the United States 1962–1989. *British Journal of Addiction*, **87**, 1345–51.

Gomberg, E. S. (1990) Drugs, alcohol, and aging. In: Kozkwski, L. T. *et al.* (eds.) *Research Advances in Alcohol and Drug Problems*, pp. 171–203. New York: Plenum Press.

Jessor, R. (1987) Problem-behaviour theory, psychosocial development and adolescent problem drinking. *British Journal of Addiction*, **82**, 331–42.

Josephson, E. and Caroll, E. E. (eds.) (1974) *Drug Use, Epidemiological and Sociological Approaches*. New York: Wiley.

Kandel, D. B. (1978) *Longitudinal Research on Drug Use*. New York: Wiley.

Kandel, D. B. (1985) On the processes of peer influences in adolescent drug use: a developmental perspective. *Advances in Alcohol and Substance Abuse*, **4**, 139–63.

Lichtenstein, P. M. (1914) Narcotic addiction. *New York Medical Journal*, **100**, 962–6.

Maddox, J. F. and Desmond, D. P. (1981) *Careers of Opioid Users*. New York: Praeger.

Mann, R. E., Smart, R., Anglin, L. and Edwards, A. (1991) Reductions in cirrhosis deaths in the United States: associations with per capita consumption and AA membership. *Journal of Studies on Alcohol*, **52**, 361–5.

McArthur, C., Waldron, E. and Dickinson, J. (1958) The psychology of smoking. *Journal of Abnormal and Social Psychology*, **56**, 267–75.

Miller, W. R. (1993) Behavioral treatments for drug problems: Where do we go from here? In: *Behavioral Treatments for Drug Abuse and Dependence*. NIDA Research Monograph **137**, pp. 303–21. Rockville, MD: National Institute on Drug Abuse.

Miller, M. A. and Kozel, N. J. (1991) *Methamphetamine Abuse: Epidemiological Issues and Implications*. NIDA Research Monograph **115**, pp. 303–21. Rockville, MD: National Institute of Drug Abuse.

Miller, W. R., Leckman, A. L., Delaney, H. D. and Tinkman, M (1992) Long-term follow-up of behavioral self-control training. *Journal of Studies on Alcohol*, **53**, 249–61.

Moos, R. H.,Mertens, J. R. and Brennan, P. L. (1993) Patterns of diagnosis and treatment among late-middle-aged and older substance abuse patients. *Journal of Studies on Alcohol*, **54**, 479–87.

O'Donnell, J. A. (1969) *Narcotic Addicts in Kentucky*. Washington DC: US Government Printing Office.

O'Donnell, J. A., Voss, H. L., Clayton, R. R., Slatin, G. T. and Room, R. G. W. (1976) *Young Men and Drugs – A Nationwide Survey*. NIDA Research Monograph **5**. Rockville, MD: National Institute on Drug Abuse.

Orford, J. and Edwards, G. (1977) *Alcoholism*. New York: Oxford University Press.

Pascarelli, E. F. (1981) Drug abuse and the elderly. In: Lowinson, J. W. and Ruiz, P. (eds.) *Substance Abuse*, pp. 752–7. Baltimore: Williams and Wilkins.

Robins, L. N. (1974) The Vietnam druguser returns. *Special Action Office Monograph Series A*, No. 2 Washington, DC: Government Printing Office.

Robins, L. N. and Regier, D. A. (1991) *Psychiatric Disorders in America*. New York: The Free Press.

Stall, R. and Biernacki, P. (1986) Spontaneous remission from the problematic use of substances: an inductive model derived from a comparative analysis of the alcohol, opiate, tobacco and food/obesity literatures. *International Journal of the Addictions*, **21**, 1–23.

Vaillant, G. E. (1966) A twelve-year follow-up of New York narcotic addicts: II The natural history of a chronic disease. *New England Journal of Medicine*, **275**, 1281–8.

Vaillant, G. E. (1968) The natural history of urban narcotic drug addiction–some determinants. In: Steinberg, H. (ed.) *Scientific Basis of Drug Dependence*, pp. 341–61. London: J. & A. Churchill.

Vaillant, G. E. (1977) *Adaptation to Life*. Boston, MA: Little Brown.

Vaillant, G. E. (1983) *Natural History of Alcholism*. Cambridge, MA: Harvard University Press.

Vaillant, G. E. (1988) What can long-term follow-up teach us about relapse and prevention of relapse in addiction? *British Journal of Addiction*, **83**, 1147–57.

Vaillant, G. E. (1993) *Wisdom of the Ego*. Cambridge, MA: Harvard University Press.

Vaillant, G. E. (1994) Evidence that the type 1/type 2 dichotomy in alcoholism must be reexamined. *Addiction*, **89**, 1049–57.

Vaillant, G. E. (1995) *Natural History of Alcoholism Revisited*. Cambridge, MA: Harvard University Press.

Weinberger, D. R. (1987) Implication of normal brain development for the pathogenesis of schizophrenia. *Archives of General Psychiatry*, **44**, 660–9.

2

Psychotherapy and the life cycle: individual and family

CHRISTOPHER DARE

Introduction

There are two groups of psychotherapies. The one that is informed by 'academic psychology' emphasises techniques that have been empirically validated by experimental procedures. The second group is that which develops using clinical thinking. The former group of therapies are mainly represented by the behavioural and cognitive psychotherapies and by combinations of the two. The second group are represented in this chapter, by reference to psychoanalytic psychotherapy and family systems thinking, although there are actually vast numbers of other therapies, humanistic, gestalt, existential and so on, which fall within this set. The first group of psychotherapies can be thought of as relying on quantitative methodology and the second upon qualitative research, although any attempt to make exclusive definitions founders. Clinical intuition cannot be precluded from any therapy and all therapies can, in principle, be validated using empirical techniques. Clinical method depends upon the use of continuous observation of patient response to inform the development of therapy in general, and with a particular patient. This is a form of empirical validation.

This chapter is about the second group of therapies: those deriving from the psychodynamic tradition in combination with family systems thinking. The additional integration of thinking from the field of child psychotherapy and family therapy, into the practice of psychotherapy, contributes resources both to the conceptual schemes and practice. Child psychotherapy demonstrates that communication does not require verbalisation. Dance therapy, music therapy and drama therapy (not to say psychodrama) are psychotherapeutic tools available for adults who, for whatever reason, cannot produce an account of their experience in words, to engage in expressive therapy. Family therapy has shown the therapeutic power of utilising the intimate social network, within which most of our patients live. This chapter recommends that those who wish to practice psychotherapy look to an expansive spectrum of practice to seek effective techniques. The author's own work, in the field of eating disorders, has shown disparate reactions to different treatments depending both on illness characteristics and such factors as age of onset and duration of illness (Dare and Crowther, 1994*a,b*; Dare and Eilser, 1994, 1995). The difference in response to treatment in different age groups of patients can be understood as a function of interactional aspects of development that constitute the family life cycle rather than as simply an age-related function.

Anything to do with psychoanalysis often appears to be retained vividly in an unchanging, anachronistic form within the minds of those mental health workers who do not see themselves primarily as psychotherapists. This can create confusion because psychoanalytic psychotherapy has changed enormously over the last quarter century. The present contribution is a rather personal account, stemming as it does from its author's interests in psychoanalytic psychotherapy for the individual and in a combined psychoanalytic and systems approach to couple and family therapy. A central theme is that psychotherapy and aetiology can be disentangled (see Dare, 1993). In the interesting psychopathological constructions that derive from both psychoanalytical and family systems models, psychogenesis need not be assumed and in this chapter a model of aetiology assuming multifactorial causes is presented. In this model, various sites and modes of psychotherapeutic intervention are proposed that can, theoretically, be effective even though 'prime causes' of the disturbance are not addressed.

The chapter begins by summarising the context from which psychoanalytic psychotherapy derives, how that set it in a certain direction, and how new ways of working have evolved. The changes in psychoanalytic thinking that need to be considered are to do with (1) developments in the psychoanalytic models of the mind and of treatment; (2) the subject matter of psychoanalysis and psychoanalytic psychotherapy; (3) the aims of psychotherapy; and (4) the modalities of treatment that are available by integration with systems thinking.

The psychoanalytic models of the mind, of symptom formation, and of therapy

A number of examples of psychoanalytic approaches to the structure of symptoms and of therapeutic interventions will be given, not to claim special privilege for them but in order to demonstrate a range of thinking and action. Psychotherapy is a task that requires access to a wide variety of techniques and skills, as the therapist crafts strategies and interventions appropriate to the task, the context and specific patient. The structure of the presentation is also historical because there is a way in which new, but also improved, versions of the same old wheel repeatedly emerge.

Figure 2.1 illustrates Freud's first model of neurosogenesis (derived from Sandler *et al.*, 1973*a*). The mind is conceived of as containing memories, important categories of which are associated with affects, portrayed in the diagram as a positive charge of emotional energy. Neurosis was thought to derive from 'an event' that is traumatic (especially sexual traumas in childhood), which could not at the origin be 'metabolised' because of the 'immaturity of the mental apparatus' (that is to say, the child was unable to grasp the full significance of the experience). Subsequently, in adolescence or adulthood the significance of the trauma was appreciated but its implications were so alarming or so socially unacceptable, that the memory had to be repressed and the affect, in consequence, was held within the mind. The power of the affect led to symptoms being developed that represented a partial release of the feelings and memories.

A particular symptom or character formation was believed to be determined by the particular mechanisms utilised to defend the person from being overwhelmed by the intensity of the retained ('strangulated') feelings, whilst the content of the memory was sometimes revealed in a symbolic symptomatic expression. An example follows.

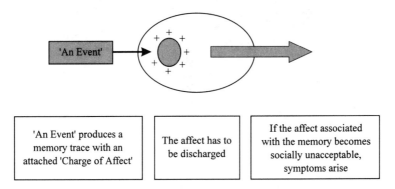

'An Event' produces a memory trace with an attached 'Charge of Affect'	The affect has to be discharged	If the affect associated with the memory becomes socially unacceptable, symptoms arise

Figure 2.1 Psychoanalytic models of the mind and of symptoms: (1) An affect-trauma model.

An elderly man presented with a long history of severe melancholia, complicated by excessive use of alcohol, drunk to deaden the pain of depression. There was a hypochondriacal element in his mental state, for he believed that some trivial skin thickening was evidence of secondary cancer. Significantly, in his history, there appeared to have been no psychiatric problems until his wife had died, relatively young and tragically of an extensive carcinoma. The melancholia had some features of morbid grief and his near-delusional belief about the skin thickening seemed an identification with his dead wife.

In this model, treatment is described as cathartic. The therapist attempts to facilitate the patient's recall of painful, past events whilst enabling ventilation of intense feelings, especially those that for personal or social reasons are particularly difficult for the patient to admit. This process is shown in Figure 2.2. Although Freud originally experimented with the use of hypnosis (e.g. Freud, 1893) to gain therapeutic catharsis, he altered his technique to one of pushing the patient to talk freely around the symptom. Freud developed the idea that he could reconstruct the memories that lay behind the symptoms by a method of interpretation of talk produced by free associations. Freud himself came to doubt the reliability of this method as a way of re-accessing lost memories. Contemporary techniques for counselling the victims of disasters, for those suffering from the death or life-threatening illness of loved ones, include an acceptance in the notion of catharsis and the benefits of full expression of the gamut of feelings aroused by painful and frightening events. The behavioural technique of forced mourning likewise contains some elements reminiscent of Freud's long-abandoned cathartic method.

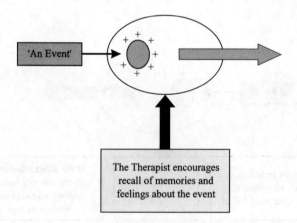

Figure 2.2 Psychoanalytic model of treatment: (1) Abreaction.

Figure 2.3 shows the archaic 'topographic model' (cf. Sandler *et al.*, 1973*b*) that Freud developed as he gave up the trauma model. This is a relatively 'closed' mental system. On the left of the figure is shown the source of the instinctual drives, the body, which impinges on the mind, demanding action. Because of the self-gratifying, ultimately selfish aim that is the essence of the drives, if their expression were to be unfettered, they would propel the individual into action that would contravene the rules of the social world. In this model, the mind evolves to balance the dual and conflicting demands of the instinctual and the social. A symptom is a disguised but disturbing expression of the mind's failure to have performed its task adequately. Drives undergo biologically determined alterations over time, so the theory has a developmental aspect. Personality formation was dominated, Freud (1905) believed, by the particular quality of the drives that had, in infancy and childhood, dominated the development of the individual.

Figure 2.4 relates the development of the symptom to this description of mental process. The arrow continuing through the ellipse labelled 'the mind' signifies the irresistible drive derivative encountering the specific social prohibition. The symptom has a meaning symbolically representing the wish, the drive that has been given content by the mind, and the opposition to that wish. The figure also attempts to illustrate that in this model, treatment is the giving of insight to the person so that the power of consciousness is mobilised against the unconscious drive demands. This version of treatment is quasi-medical, for the interpretation that creates insight was initially conceived of as almost pharmacological in

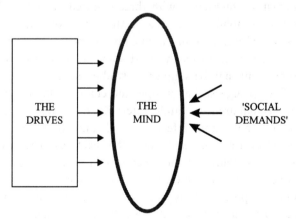

Figure 2.3 The psychoanalytic model of the mind: (2) An instinctual drive model.

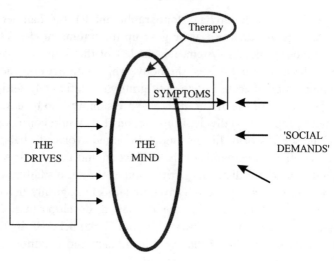

Figure 2.4 A psychoanalytic model of symptoms and therapy: (2) Interpreting the unconscious.

its qualities. Soon, Freud realised that the personal relationship that grew up between the patient and doctor was an essential source of information and a possible vehicle for treatment benefit. These ideas have become extended to create a dominant version of psychodynamic thinking. This is shown in Figure 2.5, which exemplifies a psychoanalytic object relations model.

On the left, the family of origin is portrayed. A family of two generations is shown, in interaction with three children, including the subject. This is a gross simplification, because the family of origin includes the living presence of grandparents, aunts, uncles and cousins, and the myths and legends of the ancestors. Also, at some stages of the life cycle, the main impingement may be simpler, a dyadic one dominating. Likewise, the figure fails to suggest the multiple and changing family, interactional configurations that are sequentially internalised. In addition, the presence of previous internalisations affects the style and content of future internalisations. How a person experiences the reactions of family transition at adolescence is coloured by the experience of previous transitions involving separation, for example on first going to school.

The mind is portrayed as containing multiple internalisations of interactions between others and the self and of interactions between others in the presence of the self. These patterns have a strong impact

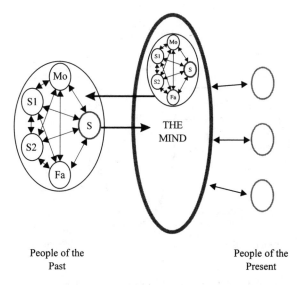

People of the
Past

People of the
Present

Figure 2.5 A psychoanalytic model of the mind: (3) An object relations model.

on establishing longed for and feared states of relationships that constitute the essential motivating structures. These have been called
'relationship needs templates' (Boszormenyi-Nagy and Spark, 1984).
They are motivating schemas within the representational world
(Sandler and Rosenblatt, 1962).

On the right-hand side of the figure is the world of contemporaries, of
the current objects. The person is in interaction with these people (as well
as having ongoing relationships with living family members). Some of the
interactions are with significant others, by which it is meant that there is a
possibility of these relationships being coloured by the inner 'relationship
needs templates'. This is a deformation, in one sense, of the 'real' relationship, a notion that is incorporated in the definition of the transference.

The idea of the symptom and of treatment is shown in Figure 2.6. The
symptom is shown, as it is theorised as existing, firmly on the boundary
between the self and the outside world. Symptomatic behaviours and
experiences may well have a symbolic meaning but they are understood
as structuring both qualities of the inner world of the person and interpersonal processes. Treatment is shown in the top right-hand side of the
figure. The person is in an intimate professional contact with the therapist, the nature of which is carefully observed by the therapist. (It is

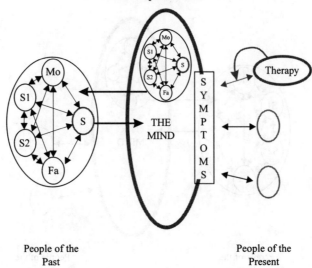

Figure 2.6 A psychoanalytic model of symptoms and therapy: (3) Interpreting the transference.

obviously difficult for a therapist to have a clear view from both sides of the interaction with the other person.) The important interventions, within this model, are those that address the multiple and complex origins of the distortions or deformations that arise in this treatment relationship. This is the analysis of the transference. In principle, this implies a belief in the efficacy of insight, but in practice contemporary psychodynamic psychotherapists are rather sceptical about the power of intellectual knowledge to promote change.

In the first half of this century, psychoanalysts had experimented with techniques to use the therapeutic relationship more forcefully and deliberately than that implied in the concept of insight promoting interpretations. The aim was to shorten the duration of psychotherapy and also to gain therapeutic efficacy in patients untouched by standard treatment. Patients with severe character problems and those who misused alcohol and drugs numbered amongst those that had prompted these experiments. Ferenczi and Rank (1925) had used techniques of getting the patient actively to oppose his or her symptomatic behaviour and had also encouraged a more dependent commitment of the patient to the therapist. Many contemporary psychoanalysts would fully agree that psychotherapeutic techniques may be much more effective if concomitant symptomatic management diminishes the addictive behaviour. This is as true in the field of eating disorder as in that of substance abuse.

Deliberate attempts to have a more permissive relationship with the patient in which regression of the patient occurs are more hazardous and controversial, as are those of the Chicago psychoanalyst Franz Alexander (Alexander and French, 1946). Alexander advocated varieties of activities on the therapist's part, whereby knowledge about transference was used to inform a rather specific stance by the psychotherapist *vis à vis* the patient. This was one in which the therapist deliberately contrived to be different from the attitudes and behaviour that characterised the parental relationship that seemed to dominate the patient's disturbance. The idea was that if the therapist could become an important figure in the patient's life and within that importance offered a style of relationship that opposed the apparently psychopathogenic influence of one or both parents, then the patient would undergo a 'corrective emotional experience'. Both Ferenczi's and Alexander's ideas of attempting to specify non-neutral patient/psychotherapist relationships remain intensely controversial. They seem plausible, and yet näive. In practice they are difficult to apply, and give rise to very intense feelings both in the patient and the therapist. In consequence they have become little used in orthodox psychoanalytic psychotherapy. The ideas appear regularly in 'new' apparently different forms of psychotherapy, especially in therapeutic residential work where professionals struggle to break into the repetitive self-destructive interpersonal behaviour of the patient.

Less controversial are ideas that can be typified as deriving from the work of the Hungarian psychoanalyst Michael Balint (1959, 1968). He developed the ideas of Sandor Ferenzci (who was both his training analyst and his teacher). Rather than suggesting a specific, long-term alteration in the psychoanalytic activity in the directions proposed by Ferenzci and Alexander, he suggested the identification of moments in therapy when the therapist should actively attempt to inaugurate change in the patient by encouraging an enactment that could foster a new beginning. The author (Dare) certainly follows this principle when he suggests, during an individual therapy, that a patient confronts a parent or a sibling about some previously unexpressed aspect of childhood relationships. Modern psychoanalysts have pointed out that psychotherapists can regularly find themselves acting in small ways that, on reflection, are slightly out of character with the therapist's usual behaviour although they may or may not be experienced as breaches of proper technique. However, on further thought, the psychoanalyst comes to see these behaviours as representing a subtle but, at the moment of action, unconscious response to aspects of the patient whose meaningfulness adds to the understanding of the patient and appears to enrich the therapeutic process. This type of reaction has been termed unconscious role responsiveness by Sandler (Sandler and Sandler, 1984) and is a useful notion for understanding certain instants in therapy and also, for the author, to understand some of the subtleties of personal relationships in many settings, especially in couple and family relationships.

In keeping with some of Balint's suggestions, Winnicott hinted at breaching the rules of abstinence in special circumstances, in the conduct of psychotherapy (holding the patient's hand was his most daring suggestion). In working with families, physical contact between therapist and young patients is possible, and at times extremely useful (accepting snotty babies on one's lap, or experiencing directly the bony emaciation of the hand and wrist of an anorexic adolescent). Modern psychoanalysts have become very interested in the quality of the therapeutic stance that they should take in response to the needs for endorsement that may be essential to initiate vulnerable, narcissistic patients into psychotherapy. However, none of these therapeutic experiments have led to a consensually agreed understanding as to the mechanism of the change that occurs in psychoanalytic psychotherapy. Nonetheless, it is believed by those of us who espouse it, to be a rather unusual therapy and that specialness can be effective in altering the inner world of object relations within the patient.

Modern object relations theory is important, for it provides a bridge between psychoanalysis and family systems notions. Family systems thinking has, at its centre, the idea that there are structures, persistent patterns of attitudes, feelings and behaviours within the intimate relationships of spouses and parents with their offspring. The model of individual development that presupposes crucial components of character organisation being built upon internalisation of the experiences within the family of origin, also proposes that acquired relationships bear the imprint of those internalisations. In practice, family and couple therapy often require more active technique than that of the dominant interpretative interventions of psychoanalytic psychotherapy, partly because the therapies tend to be brief and partly because family organisations are often robustly persistent. It is also true to say that motivation for the therapy may vary considerably in different members of the family. Activity on the part of the therapist is often necessary to make an engagement with the family or couple. Some of the experiments in more active techniques that derive within psychoanalytic psychotherapies are useful in conceptualisation of the theory of family therapy. However, it is also true to say that psychotherapy with children and adolescents has problems of motivation and engagement, as does family therapy. In both conjoint family therapy and therapy with juveniles, the therapist has to put efforts into maintaining relationships with children when the complainants are often the adults, the parents, and not the child about whom the complaints are made. It is also true that the intellectual capacity of children, and their dominant styles of thinking, makes for difficulties in 'talking about problems'. The psychoanalytic psychotherapist must find media of communication that are intellectually age-appropriate and engaging for the particular child. These technical necessities have also influenced the development of family therapies.

The subject matter of psychoanalysis and psychoanalytic psychotherapy

There is another important way in which psychotherapeutic thinking, derived from psychoanalysis, has changed over the years. This is to do with the theory of the person and of personality development. At one time, following Freud, the structure of the mind was, as mentioned above, assumed to have evolved as an organisation to contain, limit and manage instinctual drives at the behest of 'civilisation'. The imperative, unruly and intrinsically selfish sexual and aggressive instincts had to be contained, in the name of socialisation, and psychopathology was seen as a derivative of the drives finding their disguised but undisciplined expression. This theory remains in so far as the idea of unconscious but imperative wishes are believed to motivate the person. In contemporary thinking, however, these wishes derive from the historically accumulated relationship experiences in interaction with innate trends in mental life. Contemporary psychoanalytic psychotherapy takes as its subject matter these internalised experiences. They are described as 'inner objects'. In my own thinking, inner objects are mental structures, internalised representations of relationship experiences. The most inconsistent of these derive from interactions between the self and family members. Inner objects are not necessarily accurate portrayals of parents, grandparents, siblings, and so on, for experiences with such important people are worked upon and to some extent altered by fantasies and longings. It is not too much of an exaggeration to say that psychoanalytic psychotherapy is, nowadays, largely taken up with working through the crucial early family relationships, as they appear to the therapist in transference material. In this author's therapies, such psychoanalytic work resembles a form of family therapy in the absence of the family.

The aims of psychotherapy

There is another way in which the scope of thinking about psychotherapy has been widening within the psychotherapy world, under the influence of both child psychotherapy and of family systems therapy. Psychiatric treatments take as their aim the alleviation of symptoms and the reduction in an illness process. Psychoanalysis has another viewpoint, which is that treatment is aimed at something that resembles growth or personal achievement, i.e. improving the quality of health rather than the reduction of illness. However, health, like normality, is both highly subjective and necessarily socially constructed. Because most mental health professionals are adults and the highest prestige goes to those that work with people between youth and late middle-age, this age group is taken to be the paradigm of human existence. This is the group that has the financial and the electoral power and they call the shots, especially if they are additionally privileged by being white, middle-class and male. This orientation leads to some unpredictable blind spots in the development of psychotherapy techniques in mental health practice. Naturally, psychoanalytic thinking, from Freud onwards, is marked by this process.

Freud's identity as a middle-class, Jewish male living in the decades straddling the turn of the nineteenth to the twentieth century, had a clear effect on his point of view that in most ways was, naturally, invisible to him. His epigram, stating the aims of psychoanalysis, was the achievement of satisfaction in work and love. Subsequent generations of psychoanalytic psychotherapists have taken over that view without appreciating the extent to which such aims specify a person of a certain age group, at a certain level of economic security, with sufficient freedom from serious physical and psychological handicap to make both love relationships and a job possible. The definition is rather male-orientated. Until relatively recently many women, although often in paid employment outside the home, did not define themselves by their work to the same extent that it has been habitual for men so to do. However, this socially and historically determined limitation is not the main point. Freud's definition specifies an adult, who has left his family of origin sufficiently far behind, psychologically speaking, to be wishing to make his or her own love relationship with a conscious or otherwise desire to create a family.

For infants, toddlers, school-aged children and adolescents, Freud's definition is largely irrelevant, unless psychotherapists have extremely grandiose beliefs in the enduring nature of their treatments. In time, however, psychoanalysts became interested in working directly with children (as opposed to the child in the adult), and Anna Freud (1970), in particular, directed thoughts towards diffentiating the aims of treatment with children of different ages. Her formulation was in terms of libidinal development, a phraseology that comes from the belief that the psychological qualities of a particular phase of childhood were determined by the dominant quality of the sexual, sensual drives at a specific age. This is the famous sequence: oral, anal, phallic, genital, latency, adolescence and adult sexual, libidinal phases. The libidinal phases describe steps in development that coincide with directly observable changes in childhood, but the language refers to a now discredited view that the changes correspond to changes into the specific sexual energies motivating the psychology of the child. This archaicism should not be allowed to obliterate Anna Freud's achievement of identifying the aim of therapy as that of enabling the child to enter into its 'age appropriate' libidinal phase. This formulation can be understood as meaning that psychotherapy is about helping the child function socially and in relation to its own preoccupations and interests, up to its age, intelligence and physical status.

The younger contemporary of Anna Freud, Erik Erikson (1950) specified what he called an epigenetic view of development. By this he meant that each phase of development faced the person with age-specific developmental tasks, the extent to which and particular manner in which these tasks were undertaken and achieved determining the entry point and, hence, to some extent, the course of the next phase. This view of development is that which is also strongly present in Piaget's model of intellectual development. Erikson was also important in specifying a young adult, middle-age and elderly phase of the life cycle (1959). The examination of the life of Mahatma Ghandi (1970) showed that Erikson's thinking was influenced by Hindu views as to what were the life tasks of adults, and how these tasks underwent necessary changes as youth gave way to the mid-life phase. Erikson might have found comparable interests in the writings of C. G. Jung. The English Kleinian psychoanalyst Elliott Jacques (1981) drew attention, in an important paper, to the notion of 'mid-life' crisis. Without referring to Erikson, he was expressing a notion of psychological tasks that were to do with a particular phase of life, which gave qualities to that phase. Erikson and Jacques were both psychoanalysts who at the same time as maintaining an interest in the interactions between the social and the psychological, were concerned with the psychological contents of treatments. These contents are the concerns to find expression to the anxieties, pain and existential unease that characterise the adult in therapy. Gaining a sense of self-acceptance, an adequate level of self-esteem and of satisfaction with relationships, specifies the preoccupation of an adult in psychotherapy.

A contemporary approach to the aims of treatment would suggest that these tasks are an expression of attempts to succeed enough in the normal psychological tasks of that phase. These are subject to the social context of the person, are perhaps also gender determined but are also formed by the preceding psychological and physical health of the person. Once a developmental approach is firmly adopted, then treatment becomes highly subject to its imprint. Curiously, one of the dominant founding figures of family therapy Jay Haley (1973) came to a similar view as to the nature and aims of psychotherapy. He outlined a life cycle approach to therapy whereby diagnosis was not a question of identifying the presence of psychopathology but of noting the discrepancy between the person's age and location on the family life cycle. Hence, the task of a childless married couple is to find a balance betweeen the demands of personal satisfaction and commitment to the conjoint life of the couple. A couple who have established a stable style of life together become preoccupied with whether or not or when they will have a child. A child becomes an adolescent and then the family has to adapt, not to the care of a dependent child but to the presence of a potential and imminent adult. When the offspring of a family reach youthful adulthood, then the task of the family becomes that of facilitating the entry of the child into the relative social independence appropriate to that stage.

A couple were seen shortly after their oldest son, the middle of three children, had a brief psychotic episode, possibly as a result of his drink being 'spiked' wth an hallucinogen. The referring psychiatrist was alarmed at the level of conflict within the family and suggested, wisely, that if the couple could be helped with their desperate marital problem, the son's chances of further psychosis might be diminished. When seen, the couple presented as deeply miserable, blaming each other intensely for their unhappiness and insisting that he or she was unable to make things better as her or his behaviour, of which the other complained, was wholly determined by the impossible, hurtful behaviour of the other. (This is the usual quarrel as presented in marital and couple dispute, where both partners are relatively healthy.) The husband had taken to compulsive working and extremely heavy, out of control drinking after work and at the weekend. His comatose drunkenness and intense rages made him feel in the wrong, but he was, at the same time, convinced that his wife's commitment to her housework, her community, her friends and her complaints about him were the main cause of his need for his working treadmill and his drinking. For a while, the therapist could only hear the pain and despair of their complaints about each other, her unforgivingness and withdrawal, his infidelity, alcoholism and alienating fury. However, another story became visible. As a family they had been extraordinarily successful. From quite poor backgrounds, they had both been educated by their own energy and intelligence, she more than he. He however, was a financially very successful professional. They had met while young, married, had their three children, bought a large house in a fashionable suburb and had, on their own account, been completely in agreement on the upbringing of their children. At the time that the older two children were away on their tertiary education, the parents had decided to educate their youngest son at boarding school. Over the year in which he had began to live away from home in the term time, the couple had both become depressed. They realised that they had laboured on their joint family projects with the unchallenged and mutual belief that when the hard work was over they would have an idyllic life in a long retirement. What happened was the reverse. She felt desperately lonely and isolated. He was exhausted, irritated with their friends (actually exclusively drawn from her social contacts), disappointed sexually, wanting to move the location of his work (it was his own business). His previously heavy social drinking became a dominant fact in his life. He began an affair with a family friend. In couple work they both realised how little realism had been in their plans, how much they had assumed that the other was the reason for their existence, and how little they were able to work out what they really wanted for themselves. On a developmental, life cycle assessment, the problem that was unearthed by their son's breakdown was the rigidity with which the family had been decided as an organisation within which the parents dedicated themselves to their children. When the children were launched on their own lives, the parents (and, as it turned out, the children) believed that the family was defunct. When parents 'live for their children' the absence of children can be a dangerous crisis.

Adults, living in relative separation from the family from whence they have come, will be making decisions about what style of life is right for them, and about what sort of social relationships they wish to be with. Psychological casualty can be defined in terms of a difficulty in moving from one style of age-determined relationship to the next phase.

The life cycle, the individual and therapy

A general proposition concerning the choice of psychotherapeutic strategy can be drawn: The more a person is involved in a family of origin or a family of creation, the more possible it is that some form of conjoint, couple or marital therapy will not only be possible but advantageous. The more a person is detached from both family of origin and family of creation, the more the focus of treatment will be upon the patient alone. The aim of therapy does not change with the modality; the social context, the people in the consulting room in which that aim is sought, does.

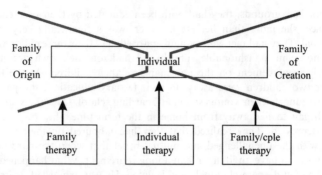

Figure 2.7 The life cycle, the individual and therapy.

Figure 2.7 illustrates this account. The open trapezium on the left represents the family of origin, existing before the subject, the individual, and enclosing this person entirely in infancy. Of course, the blunt end of the trapezium does not imply that the family of origin comes to the end of its existence, when the person leaves home. The middle section of the rectangle, representing the individual, presupposes that in young adulthood there is a period of relative psychological independence marked in many affluent societies by a period of physical independence, at college, travelling, doing military service or simply working and living with a peer group in a flat or lodgings. People who do not leave home, physically, in this phase of the life-cycle, may or may not be having a problem of psychological separation. It is a crisis, in the specialist sense of this chapter, a time when a large number of psychiatric conditions become evident. It is likely that the development of psychiatric disturbance at this time makes the separation difficult. However, it is also useful to see that the crisis of this phase can be a major precipitant of a psychiatric breakdown, the form of which may be both socially and constitutionally determined.

The trapezium on the right side of the diagram represents the family of creation, beginning with the coming together of the couple, who then usually have children. A lot of psychotherapy occurs around the problem of couple formation and in the maintenance of the couple. Psychotherapy for the individual often seems to me to be a way of coping with and sometimes of avoiding exploration of the problems of the couple. Psychiatry has a view that women are more often properly designated as the patient. Many would be sceptical of this tendency. It is a masculine convenience to believe that a couple problem is caused by the woman's neuroticism, her depression or her tranquillizer dependence. This view relieves men from looking at their problem of providing appropriate nurturance and support for families with young children. This issue reaches crisis point during the phase when the couple are pregnant and have infants and toddlers to care for. The problems that families have at this stage are called depression in the woman but have been shown to be strongly associated with the lack of a supportive relationship (see Brown and Harris, 1978). It must be made quite clear that substituting a diagnosis of a marital problem for an individual psychopathology is not what is being advocated. Seeing the relationship dimension increases the range of treatment possibilities, not a widening of the possibility of sickness attributions.

During the course of family life, crises occur around the addition or loss of family members or the threat of loss or addition. These crises are potent life events, initiators of psychological distress and psychiatric breakdown. Without these almost universally experienced but not inevitable life events, there are the crises that are bound, in any case, to occur, imposed by the transitions in the life cycle. Like the trapezium on the left, representing the family of creation, the open trapezium on the right of the figure comes to enclose the individual; the crises become family transitions. The crises come about in the course of the demand for mutually responsive psychological changes to each other and for each other that people must make in order that the family 'works' for the evolving and different needs of all the family members. Because change requires mutual adaptation, family or couple focused interventions are strategies that might be useful alternatives or additions to individually orientated treatments. Symptoms, whatever they are or whatever their origins, in the model being presented, are examined in the context of identifying what crises the family has gone through and towards which the breakdown is, amongst other causative and precipitating factors, a response. Another way of saying the same thing, is that a full diagnostic formulation inquires as to which family transitions are being slowed or avoided by the appearance of breakdown in an individual at such crises.

Somewhere on the right-hand side of Figure 2.7, there is a point at which the children of the family of creation reach adolescents. This usually coincides with (or precipitates) a mid-life reappraisal by one or both parents, as in the couple described above. Of course, biological changes (for example, middle-age illness, or the menopause) may have contributed to the onset of this reappraisal. The coincidence of individual transitions in more than one generation can intensify the crises for the family. Involutional breakdown in a parent generation or depression in an old person of the grandparent generation, may all be seen as part of a crisis occurring in the three-generational organisation.

Couple and family therapy

There is no space to describe the wide range of techniques that can be used in couple and family therapy. What is emphasised is that, in dealing directly with family or partnership interactions, the subject matter of conjoint treatments is not extraordinarily different from that of modern psychodynamic psychotherapy with individuals. Symptoms are treated as though they simultaneously exist and function within the individual and between individuals (which is essentially a derivative of the transference notions of modern object relations theory). Couple and family therapy seek to find the power to challenge and demote the symptom within these extant personal relationships, rather than to seek the establishment of a special relationship between the patient and therapist, to achieve therapeutic leverage. Although the means chosen to achieve therapeutic movement differ markedly in conjoint as opposed to individual psychodynamic psychotherapy, the means of achieving change may have unforseen convergence.

It is being suggested that although symptoms add serious handicap and disadvantage to the life of the person, they also have a function, for example, by modulating demands for change during life cycle transitions. This is certainly a psychodynamic formulation, implying that symptoms have function as well as meaning. However, it must be reiterated that the meaning and function accruing to symptoms can be seen as occurring along the side of or after the symptom's arrival rather than having the specific capacity to create the symptoms. Because a symptom or illness appears to have a psychological function for the individual (or the couple or family), there need be no aetiological implication. Something that turns out to be a convenience does not have to be psychologically caused. Individuals do not invent the heroin or alcohol that they use. The substances are, literally or figuratively, acquired on the street. Having been found, and given whatever it takes, physically speaking, to become addicted, the substance use then becomes a fact of psychological life that can become incorporated into defensive mechanisms or character organisations. The addiction or habituation can become used for the enactment of fantasies and the control of affects such as interpersonal anxieties. The use to which the substance is put is not an origin or source of the substances.

Modern psychotherapeutic thinking requires a complex model of the origin of symptoms and of psychological illness. Such a complex model also implies a range of locations in the complex, interacting causative, maintaining and modifying multiple factors where therapy might occur. A suggestion for an aetiological diagram is offered in Figure 2.8. Genetic and social causes of symptoms are shown at the top of the figure. The arrow leading to the symptom is shown as unidirectional, implying that the existence of the symptoms in the person has influence neither on the social context nor on the genetic constitution of the person. Likewise, the genetic make-up and the social structures impinge on all the individual members of the family. A large, powerful and famous extended family may have some influence in shaping certain aspects of their culture, but this is unusual. Unidirectional arrows are shown connecting social and cultural influences on the individual people of the family. There are definite societal influences that have direct bearing on many structural features of the family as a system. The family and the individual are shown as a mutually interacting, bidirectional structure.

The symptom (which can be organised in and by a psychological illness) is shown in interaction with the individual and the family as a whole. The concept of the life cycle is shown as an ellipse, overlapping with social and genetic factors, which strongly influence its course. The life cycle is also shown as enclosing the individual and the family, structuring as it does the course of life and the interaction between the individual and the family, and all other relationships. The main point of this presentation is the interaction between the symptom and the life cycle.

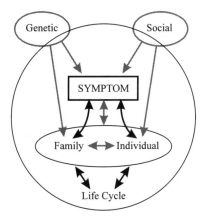

Figure 2.8 Aetiology and the dynamics of the life cycle.

The symptom, having arisen from whatever cause or group of interacting causes, becomes interposed between the individual, the family and other social relationships and has a profound affect on the life course. The symptoms then gain the meaning and functionality referred to before, which at worst fixes the person in the stage of the life cycle at which the symptom commenced. It has been remarked, for example, that some dependent opiate users seem to remain stuck in a style, a pattern of life that pertained at the time of first using the drug. When observing conjoint therapy meetings with adult opiate users, I have been strongly impressed by the easygoing comfort of the group, appearing much like a family at ease with pre-adolescent offspring. A 35-year-old, 20 years into her anorexia, complained that she was still financially dependent on her parents and she could not yet foresee a time when she would be able to leave home. We are all familiar with the middle-aged man with schizophrenia, going around with his aged parents like an 11-year-old child.

The range of applicability of psychotherapies, and the widening scope of psychotherapy

The previous section argued that contemporary psychodynamic psychotherapy has widened the range of conditions for which it can be applied; there have been profound alterations in the model of the mind, its development and the nature of psychopathology. This leads to modification of the type of change that is sought in psychotherapy. The psychodynamic model can also utilise some of the conceptual models of family systems thinking in order to contribute a yet wider range of treatment possibilities.

Figure 2.9 relates the preceding aetiological and life cycle diagram to psychotherapeutic strategies. The customary conceptualisation of the psychotherapies has seen them as addressed to theoretical psychogenetic hypotheses. This is shown in Figure 2.9 by the grey arrows ascending from the bottom of the diagram and impinging upon the family (on the left) or the individual (on the right). These imply the notion, respectively, of a conjoint family therapy that seeks to correct a supposed family cause for a problem or an individual psychotherapy aimed at addressing suggested individual psychological causes. The horizontal grey arrows postulate alternative strategies, namely those that are directed towards processes interposed between the symptom and the individual or the symptom and the family. This suggests therapies that are not necessarily seeking to alter primary causes of a disorder but, rather, to tackle the individual psychological or family processes that contribute to the development, or, equally, the maintenance of a symptom. The theoretical model of therapy is an alternative to the idea that psychological or family processes give rise to symptoms (although such aetiologies exist). It proposes that, once having arisen, symptoms come to play a part in the psychological organisation of the individual or the family. Psychotherapy attempts to undo the role that the symptoms have come to assume in the psychological structuring of the individual or the family.

Alternatively, therapy might seek to disarticulate social processes impinging on the individual (the shorter, grey arrow on the right) and participating in the generation of the symptom. What is in mind here are, for example, attempts to separate an adolescent from participation in a street culture that puts the person at risk of continuing substance abuse, or whatever.

Figure 2.9 poses the possibility of choosing diverse and complementary strategies based upon empirical evaluation rather than the advocacy of a particular 'brand name' psychotherapy linked to a specific psychopathological theory.

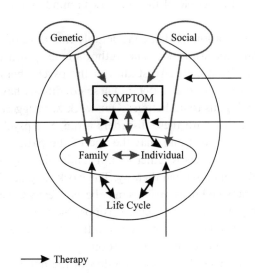

Figure 2.9 Aetiology, therapy and the dynamics of the life course.

Christopher Dare

Conclusions

Psychoanalytic psychotherapy can be freed from the demand that it deals with fundamental causes by being agnostic about the relationship between aetiology and psychopathology. The aim of therapy has thus moved from the idea of correcting a supposed underlying psychological structure towards that of demoting the interaction between symptom, psychopathology and the achievement of a move in the life cycle. Further, the life cycle is defined as, inevitably, including the person absorbed to a lesser or greater extent in a close psychological network; a family or something like a family. Psychotherapy can only proceed without regard to the psychological matrix of the personal network, under special circumstances, that is, in the young adult phase. For social reasons, working with this group has high prestige and has been seen as the paradigm for all therapy. This has created an artefact that has obscured the need to consider other life cycle phases and transitions in psychotherapeutic work. This can often be addressed effectively by working directly with the personal relationship network that is in couple or family work. Work with the network can be indirect, that is with the relationship with the people of the network in mind, without their literal presence.

All these considerations widen considerably the range of psychoanalytic psychotherapeutic strategies. The author's main justification for the assertions comes from extensive studies in the psychotherapy of eating disorders (see Szmukler *et al.*, 1995). These conditions have themselves been seen as analogous to addictions. Our work has suggested that there is some evidence that with these disorders a range of psychotherapeutic strategies can be effective and that the age of the patient at which the disturbance began predicts whether or not family therapy is more likely to be successful than individual therapy. The work suggests that attention to the world of personal relationships may be as effective, therapeutically, as a more purely symptomatic focus. It is possible to make interventions based upon the psychodynamic interpretation but using structural or strategic modes as well as by interpretation.

The move away from drive-based models of the mind, to those based on object relations theory or self psychology, has led to psychoanalytic psychotherapy being directed towards transference interpretations. In consequence, these individual therapies resemble family therapy without the family. Psychotherapy with couples has been shown to be more likely to benefit the couple relationship than does separate, individual therapy with both halves of the couple (Gurman and Kniskern, 1981). It is not known (because the studies have not be conducted) whether or not this outcome distinction would be shown to be true when the target is more individual and symptom-orientated as opposed to relationship-focused. In the few available relevant studies of separated as opposed to conjoint family therapy, it can be shown that seeing the family members separately can produce as good or even better results than with conjoint work (see Szapocznik, 1986; Szapocznik and Kurtines, 1989; Le Grange *et al.*, 1992*b*). In our studies on eating disorder, the targets of therapy have been symptoms not relationships. Indeed, our own rather sparse data suggest that family therapy with adolescent eating disorder patients is more successful in those families whose relationships are relatively harmonious at the beginning of therapy, with scanty evidence that the family therapy has an important effect on improving family satisfaction (Le Grange *et al.*, 1992*a*). The small body of research on the psychotherapy and family therapy of substance abuse (e.g. Stanton *et al.*, 1982; Woody *et al.*, 1983; Szapocznik and Kurtines, 1989) illustrate the possibility of usefulness for the analogies between eating disorders and addictions that are being drawn upon in this chapter. The principles outlined, which have proved useful in the field of eating disorder, may be helpful with patients misusing substances.

Acknowledgement

The author gratefully acknowledges the support given to the work reported here by the Trustees of the Bethlem Royal and Maudsley Hospital, the Medical Research Council of Great Britain, and the Leverhulme Foundation.

References

Alexander, F. and French, T. M. (1946) *Psychoanalytic Therapy*. New York: Ronald Press.
Balint, M. (1959) *Thrills and Regression*. London: Hogarth.
Balint, M. (1968) *The Basic Fault*. London: Tavistock Publications.
Boszormenyi-Nagy, I. and Spark, G. (1984) *Invisible Loyalties: Reciprocity in Intergenerational Family Therapy*. New York: Harper Row.
Brown, G. W. and Harris T. (1978) *Social Origins of Depression: A Study of Psychiatric Disorder in Women*. London: Tavistock.
Dare, C. (1993) Aetiological models and the psychotherapy of psychosomatic disorders. In: Hodes, M. and Morey, S. (eds.) *Psychotherapy and Psychosomatic States*, pp. 9–29. London: Gaskill Publications.

Dare, C. and Crowther, C. (1994*a*). Psychodynamic models of eating disorders. In: Szmukler, G., Dare, C. and Treasure, J. (eds.) *Eating Disorders; Handbook of Theory, Treatment and Research*, pp. 125–140. Chichester: John Wiley.

Dare, C. and Crowther, C. (1994*b*). Living dangerously: psychoanalytic psychotherapy of eating disorder. In: Szmukler, G., Dare, C. and Treasure, J. (eds.) *Eating Disorders: Handbook of Theory, Treatment and Research*, pp. 275–92. Chichester: John Wiley.

Dare, C. and Eisler, I. (1994). Family therapy. In: Szmukler,G., Dare, C. and Treasure, J (eds.) *Eating Disorders; Handbook of Theory, Treatment and Research*. pp. 333–50, Chichester: John Wiley.

Dare, C. and Eisler, I. (1995) Family therapy. In: Kelly, K. D. and Fairburn, C. (eds.) *Comprehensive Textbook of Eating Disorder and Obesity*. New York: Oxford Publications (in press).

Erikson, E. H. (1950) *Childhood and Society*. New York: Norton.

Erikson, E. H. (1959) Identity and the life cycle. *Psychological Issues Monograph*, **1**. New York: International Universities Press.

Erikson, E. H. (1970) *Ghandi's Truth: On the Origins of Militant Non-Violence*. London: Faber.

Ferenczi, S. and Rank, O. (1925) *The Development of Psychoanalysis*. New York: The Nervous and Mental Diseases Publishing Co.

Freud, A. (1970) Child analysis as a subspeciality of psychoanalysis. In: *The Writings of Anna Freud*, vol. 7, pp. 204–19. London: Hogarth Press.

Freud, S. (1893) A case of successful treatment by hypnosis. In: Strachey, J. (ed.) *The Standard Edition of the Complete Psychological Works of Sigmund Freud*, vol. 1. London: Hogarth Press.

Freud, S. (1905) Three essays on the theory of sexuality. In: Strachey, J. (ed.) *The Standard Edition of the Complete Psychological Works of Sigmund Freud*, vol. 7, pp. 125–243. London: Hogarth Press.

Gurman, A. S. and Kniskern, D. P. (1981) Family therapy outcome research: knowns and unknowns. In: Gurman, A. S. and Kniskern, D. P. (eds.) *Handbook of Family Therapy*, pp. 742–75. New York: Brunner/Mazel.

Haley, J. (1973) *Uncommon Therapy: The Psychiatric Techniques of Milton H. Erickson, M.D.* New York: Grune & Stratton.

Jacques, E. (1981) The midlife crisis. In: Greenspan, S. I. and Pollock, G. H. (eds.) *The Course of Life. Volume 3: Adulthood and the Aging Process*, pp. 1–23. Washington: US DHHS.

Le Grange, D., Eisler, I., Dare, C. and Hodes, M. (1992*a*) Family criticism and self starvation: a study of expressed emotion. *Journal of Family Therapy*, **14**, 177–92.

Le Grange, D., Eisler, I., Dare, C. and Russell, G. F. M. (1992*b*) Evaluation of family therapy in anorexia nervosa: a pilot study. *International Journal of Eating Disorder*, **12**, 347–5

Sandler, J., Holder, A. and Dare, C. (1973*a*) Frames of reference in psychoanalytic psychology. IV. The affect-trauma frame of reference. *British Journal of Medical Psychology*, **45**, 265.

Sandler, J., Holder, A. and Dare, C. (1973*b*) Frames of reference in psychoanalytic psychology. V. The topographical frame of reference: The organization of the mental apparatus. *British Journal of Medical Psychology*, **46**, 29.

Sandler, J. and Rosenblatt, B. (1962) The concept of the representational world. *The Psychoanalytic Study of the Child*, **18**, 139–158.

Sandler, J. and Sandler, A. M. (1984) The past unconscious, the present unconscious, and interpretation of the transference. *Psychoanalytic Inquiry*, **4**, 367–99.

Stanton, M. D., Todd, T. C. and Associates (1982) *The Family Therapy with Drug Abuse and Addiction*. New York: Guilford.

Szapocznik, J. (1986) Conjoint versus one-person family therapy: further evidence for the effectiveness of conducting family therapy through one person with drug-abusing adolescents. *Journal of Consulting and Clinical Psychology*, **54**, 395–7.

Szapocznik, J. and Kurtines, W. M. (1989) *Breakthroughs in Family Therapy with Drug Abusing and Problem Youth*. New York: Springer.

Szmukler, G., Dare, C. and Treasure J. (eds.) (1995) *Handbook of Eating Disorders: Theory, Treatment and Research*. Chichester: Wiley.

Woody, G. E., Luborsky, L., McLellan, A. T. *et al.* (1983) Psychotherapy for opiate addiction: Does it work? *Archieves of General Psychiatry*, **40**, 639–45.

3

Personal strengths and vulnerability in family and social context

GILL GORELL BARNES

Introduction

This chapter will consider some of the social and family factors that create a stressful context for children growing up. The impact of life events as additional stressors is discussed. There is no attempt to put this together with the abuse of drugs, which is attended to elsewhere in the book. However, the relationship between social disadvantage, stressful life events, and the recourse to drugs will be apparent to many readers.

As discussed in Chapter 7 a systemic approach to treatment is one that considers problems in the context both of intimate relationships and of the wider social network of which an individual is a part. The intimate relationships within which a young person exists have a developmental aspect, and a life span perspective. This means that the social boundaries relevant to the growing child will constantly be in change. Society will also place demands for change relating to culture, class and race. Gender will in addition create widely differing expectations in relation to role within the family (Gorell Barnes, 1995).

Using a systemic lens, four broad principles for looking at the connection between individuals and families may be useful.

1. People in families are intimately connected, and focusing on those connections can be a more valid way to understand and promote change in problem-related behaviour than focusing on the perspective of any one individual.
2. People living in close proximity over time set up patterns of interaction made up of relatively stable sequences of interaction.
3. The patterns of interaction, belief, and behaviour that therapists observe and address can be understood both as cause and effect of the problem: the 'fit' between the problem and the family.

44

4. Problems within patterns of family life are related to inappropriate adaptation to some environmental influence or change, either realised or anticipated (Gorell Barnes and Cooklin, 1994).

Mutual influence and family life

In the last decade much research into family life and the onset of different forms of psychological illness has explored the impact of stressful life events in terms of the *meanings* that these events are given by individuals, and the impact of these meanings on subsequent choices of relationship (Dohrenwend and Dohrenwend, 1984; Brown *et al.*, 1986; Brown, 1990, 1991; Harris *et al.*, 1990). Patterns of childhood deprivation and the attribution of negative meaning to subsequent life events may predispose to continuity of *negative* experience within the lifetime of an individual or between the generations. However, these and other studies (Quinton and Rutter, 1984; Rutter, 1987, 1990) have also looked at how former patterns of deprivation can be changed by subsequent intimate relationships. Such studies provide evidence on a broader scale for the clinical hypothesis that what people believe on the basis of their former life experience, is intimately connected to their current overall well-being, to the choices they make, and to their capacity to respond with resilience or helplessness in the face of fresh life stress.

There are a wide variety of adverse experiences that children can go through in the course of their developing lives. Some of these combine and amplify one another. Some are rooted within the individual child, others within family members, especially the parents, while others reflect poor socio-economic status. The way in which life expectations can be adversely affected by economics, by deprived urban surroundings, by poor housing and disadvantaged, marginalised peer groups, is likely to be well-known to all those who work with young people addicted to drugs.

Long-term effects of family experience

The long-term effect of family patterns, whether positive or negative, is obviously a question of great importance to all professionals who work with families and have the aim of intervening in systems contributing to problems in children. Maccoby (1980) has argued that the main effect of family experience on social development is not the learning of specific behaviours for children growing up, but instead the lasting influences that come from the establishment of modes of interaction with other people; patterns of feeling, thinking and behaving; and from the acquisition of particular patterns of adaptation to changing life circumstances. She is thus arguing for the concept of children learning patterns or principles of relating, rather than just 'behaviours'. These patterns have effects on self-concept, on processes of identification, and on the development of a sustained pattern of social interaction. In particular, dysfunction develops in relation to aggression, quarrelling and inability to set up mechanisms within the family for problem solving (Rutter, 1984; Cummings, 1987; Emery, 1989; Jenkins and Smith, 1990; Patterson and Capaldi, 1990).

The carry forward of pattern

What contributes to the carry forward of pattern? Conversely, where the pattern is adverse, what are the protective factors that, in buffering against stress, may allow sufficient flexibility for new patterns to develop (Radke-Yarrow and Sherman, 1990)?

Two studies that give evidence for the idea of family-system characteristics carried forward through the generations are those of Belsky and Pensky (1988), and Caspi and Elder (1988). Belsky and Pensky consider the evidence relating to child maltreatment, spouse abuse and marital instability, and look at the acquisition process by which young children relate to positive and negative adult interactions. They use the concept of **internal working models** (Bowlby, 1980; Bretherton, 1985; Maine *et al.*, 1985; Sroufe and Fleeson, 1988). Internal working models are defined as affectively laden mental representations of the self, other and of the relationships derived from interactional experiences. These models function outside conscious awareness to direct attention and organise memory in ways that guide interpersonal behaviour and interpretation of social experience. The active role of the individual in interpreting the experienced world, and the inclination to assimilate information into pre-existing models, means that interpersonal development is likely to be conservative. The individual is likely to disregard inconsistent information or to reinterpret it.

Sroufe and Fleeson (1988), also using the concept of internal working models, have suggested that it is the pattern as a whole, the 'representation of relationship', that is learnt by the child. Represented relationships are carried forward. In studying children who have been abused as they move into subsequent relationship contexts, they observed that children can replay the position of the abused or the abuser relationship. They assert that relationship systems as wholes have continuity and coherence, that the whole system is reflected in each sub-relationship and that entire representational systems are carried forward. As an assertion, this has powerful implications for family patterns that change within a child's lifetime, and bears out clinical experience of the reproduction or re-enactment of former family pattern in families that have separated and then remarried.

In addition, the question of why some people are more affected by stressful experience or distressing life events than others who have had comparable experience has been studied over the last 15 years. Certain positive dimensions in family life are shown to be of primary importance. These include a good parenting bond for the later self-esteem of women and mothers; the importance of an intimate peer relationship for women who are mothers with a young child; the value of a good marital relationship in repairing earlier deprivation and contributing to good parenting. In addition, certain qualities of family life contribute to the well-being of children: communication that is relatively free from aggression and the capacity to allow appraisal of stressful situations.

Emde (1988), in thinking about the relevance of research to clinical intervention, addresses the question of individual meaning and the way in which lived experience becomes transformed into represented relationships. How do repeated interactions influence the formation of represented relationships, which include ways of looking at the world, affective themes and social-value systems? In addition, how do configurational patterns, begun in families, couple with other social systems with which the family interact? Do these offer the opportunity for more flexible development and variety in options, or do they become more stereotypic in their transaction with the family? At which points do children's ways of viewing the world become relatively inflexible and self-perpetuating? When do rare events (trajectories or random factors) lead to new learning within systemic patterns (Quinton and Rutter, 1984; Rutter, 1990; Radke-Yarrow and Sherman, 1990)?

The sections that follow briefly outline three areas of social disadvantage that may place children and young people at additional risk. These are acute social disadvantage, mental illness and family breakup. The orientation is primarily that of a clinician who is interested in what research shows us may be useful to our thinking and to our daily work. The intention is to relate research to ongoing questions relating to the family. How do these factors affect intimacy and attachment or connectedness; what promotes resilience in the family; and what are the protective features in any one family that are likely to protect children in spite of the adverse circumstances?

Poverty and family life

Recent figures on poverty in the UK reveal the imbalance of economic power between men and women, both inside marriage and without (Henwood *et al.*, 1987; Glendinning and Millar, 1987). Women are significantly poorer than men throughout Europe (Boh *et al.*, 1989). Women maintain care-giving systems for children, and for elderly and dependent members of the family. Awareness of the changing marriage patterning and the effect on family life through the growth of lone, female-headed families in the UK has drawn attention to wider issues of the feminisation of poverty. While 16% of all UK families are lone parent-headed this figure rises as high as 32% in some inner city areas (Kiernan and Wicks, 1990). Lone parents are unlikely to rise from the poverty trap (Cook and Watts, 1987). Structural inequalities of this kind therefore need to form an important part of the awareness of all who attempt to work with families who may have developed particular forms of adaptation and resilience in response to the survival skills that poverty requires. These may include drug trafficking in various forms. The question of how drug use is linked to relationship expectations and maintenance will be referred to below.

The Newcastle Study (Kolvin *et al.*, 1988 *a,b,c*), indicates that the three key risk factors for children are poor mothering, overcrowding and marital disruption. The study also demonstrated that cumulative risk changes in response to change in social milieu. When deprivation increased over time, so did social offending; when it decreased, so did the subsequent rates of criminality.

This list is remarkably similar to one compiled from the research of Rutter and his colleagues. Cumulative disadvantage is drawn from the following six variables: severe marital discord, low social status, overcrowding or large family size, paternal criminality, maternal psychiatric disorder, the placement of a child in the care of local authority.

A child with only one of these risk factors fared almost as well as did children with none. The presence of two risk factors increased the probability of disorder fourfold. Among children with four or more risk factors, 21% had manifest problems (Rutter, 1978, 1979, 1984, 1985, 1987).

Ethnicity and culture

There has until recently been a reluctance to document patterns of survival and patterns of breakdown in families from different ethnic groups, in case such documentation could be construed as racial prejudice. However, considering the distribution of different ethnic and cultural groups within all societies, it would seem appropriate rather than discriminatory for researchers to include distinctions and differences in belief systems as part of their enquiry (Stone, 1988; Hardy, 1994). Recently, black professionals themselves have become more vocal about the need for white professionals to recognise ethnic differences in addition to distinctions created by racist practices. White professionals have been urged to take a structural pluralist view of society that acknowledges there are many perspectives of reality of equal validity. The logical consequences may be in conflict with one another (Fernando, 1991). The attempt to construct a homogeneous view of reality in an approach to social issues that have discrete racial and cultural nuances may disqualify the experience as well as the strengths of black families of different ethnicities, especially when the inequalities of structure and power currently built into society are ignored. The meaning of participating in drug-related activities and the relationship of these to family and gendered values and beliefs will be important to deconstruct among different groups of young people, rather than assuming that there are meanings common to all.

The impact of mental illness

In considering the impact of parental illness on children, the factors that buffer children against stressful experience in many other contexts have relevance also. Chronic adversity, in distinction from mild adversity, implies acute or erratic and unpredictable onset, moderate to high intensity and ongoing duration. Some children's lives will be lived in the context of interactions that are framed by this quality of experience. Interparental conflict, violence or inappropriate abusive behaviour towards the child, may all occur when the child is not perceived as a child or as a developmentally dependent being in the process of growth and change, but is construed as a 'fixed object' against which certain kinds of personal and interpersonal phenomena are directed. Maternal psychiatric disorder may be of particular difficulty for the child if the father is not prepared to act as an alternate intimate and safe base. Cumulative risk for the child might include mental illness in either parent combined with high maternal anxiety or rigidity in attitudes and belief systems with regard to the child's development. Such attitudes are especially disadvantageous where they contain prejudices or perceptions likely in themselves to harm development, such as the belief that the child carries malign intentions towards the parent (Downey and Coyne, 1990; Garmezy and Masten, 1994). Where there are few positive parental interactions, attention may need to be paid to additional protection from outside the family.

In a wider systemic context, such factors will be likely to be increased by poverty, large family size and reduced family support from any extended family. Stressful life events will further contribute to hazards for the family's functioning (Samaroff and Seifer, 1990). In citing factors that have been found in research to amplify the adverse effects of mental illness, it becomes difficult to tease out which factors relate to social disadvantage and which factors to mental illness. As in any other overall appraisal of the appropriate level for potential family intervention, the clinician always needs to bear in mind other correlates of mental illness such as job insecurity or unemployment, and the effect of these on family relationships. This is now referred to as comorbidity in studies of risk (Garmezy and Masten, 1994). Resilience factors of value to the child emerge from earlier studies of Rutter (1979), Sameroff and Seifer (1990) and Kolvin (1988a). These include the presence of a second parent in the home and an understanding of the relationship episodes that maintain the child's own positive self concept. These may include regular interactions with a reliable adult outside the home whom the child can talk to, the value of ongoing peer groups through school or sport, and a reliable and continuing social life that includes the opportunity to play and to maintain a child's world away from the home milieu (Gorell Barnes *et al.*, 1995).

Parental mental disorder and the effect on children

The emphasis on a single risk factor often camouflages other common effects of mental illness, which include poverty, job insecurity or unemployment, being on state benefit, marital instability, marital discord and negative child-rearing practices. Thus research is now giving support to the thinking, long-held by social workers and other non-medical professionals, that it is less useful to attempt to attribute problems of children of mentally ill parents to a specific factor, rather than to aspects of the fit between the illness and the social surround in which it is lodged.

Similarities in the behaviour patterns of children across different forms of mental illness may relate more to inadequate or malignant parenting and negative psychosocial similarities.

Children of criminal parents

Risk factors for delinquencies implicate genetics, physiological processes (hyperactivity, etc.), educational failure, overcrowded slum housing, high crime neighbourhood, drug availability, and all the negative family patterns already discussed.

Protective factors

Protective factors that may shield children in many of the circumstances outlined above include the following (Garmezy, 1985, 1987; Rutter, 1985, 1987, 1990; Kolvin *et al.*, 1988*a*; Masten *et al.*, 1990):

(i)   adequate job opportunities
(ii) educational opportunities (school attendance, positive peer group influence, school leadership, demands for achievement, positive efforts by teachers)
(iii) community (available social services, low neighbourhood delinquency rates, movement away from high delinquency rates)
(iv) family factors (cohesiveness, maternal and paternal love, consistent discipline, parental supervision, positive parental marital relationship, home ownership, parental stability)

Divorce

Divorce now affects one in four children in the UK before the age of 16 (Kiernan and Wicks, 1990). Recent analysis of cohort data (Elliot and Richards, 1991) has shown how the disruptive effect of parental quarrelling and unhappiness can be seen to affect children's performance in school and their emotional well-being some years before a divorce takes place (see also Jenkins and Smith, 1990). Research on the impact of divorce therefore cannot answer the question of how these children would have fared had their parents stayed together. Divorce alone cannot be seen as a risk factor independent of the social effects and emotional interactions in which it is embedded.

Gorell Barnes (1991*a*) has reviewed some of the divorce literature that shows the multiple pathways followed by children and families after divorce, and the differences in family pattern that need to be attended to by professionals. These include: (1) the health of the family in the early stage of reorganisation, and awareness that mothers will be experiencing higher stress and reduced income (Guidobaldi and Cleminshaw, 1985); (2) the reduction of quarrelling between parents in the post-divorce access situation as an important factor in the maintenance of the child's self-esteem (Lund, 1987); (3) the importance of supportive networks for lone parents; (4) clarifying communication with the child about processes in the family and relationships with absent parents (Mitchell, 1985; Gorell Barnes, 1991*b*).

A number of researchers have distinguished between marked but transient symptomatic behaviour in children following the decision to divorce, and longer-term difficulties. Hetherington (1989) has pointed out the diversity of children's responses. Many children show remarkable resilience and develop enhanced coping mechanisms. Others sustain developmental delay or show delayed effects. There are marked gender differences in children's responses both to divorce and remarriage (Zazlow, 1988*a,b*). The degree to which the coherence of a former family pattern, now dissolved by divorce, may be carried forward into new family situations is not one that is established on a research basis. Concepts from child development studies such as the carrying forward of patterns of relationship or internal working models (Sroufe and Fleeson, 1988), are valuable in understanding why families who have formed new structures may appear to repeat previous patterns that were performed and had their meaning in former family lives.

Lone-parent and extended family structures

Lone-parent families consist of two major groups: the never-married mother and the post-cohabitation or post-divorce lone-parent family. The second group forms the largest group in the UK. Never-married mothers form a small percentage of households, most of which are of short duration. Nearly 30% of first births are to unmarried women. The family patterns that they subsequently develop are various. The meaning of lone parenthood will differ depending on the cultural background of the woman who bears children without a partner. However, certain key factors will affect all lone parents such as the lack of financial security, the difficulty of earning an adequate income as well as rearing children, and the ways in which definitions of relationship between men who form a transient or semi-permanent part of the household and the children who rely on a long-term stable relationship with the mother, are maintained. In working with lone-parent families it is important to consider wider supportive networks of which they may be a part, and to consider kinship as well as friendship systems that may provide important intimate networks for women.Where these are lacking, the creation of support systems through such projects as Newpin (Mills *et al.*, 1984), may be an important part of work with the family. The stress that a small family system can manage may be improved by better connections with wider social systems.

Step-families

Step-families can be formed in a wide variety of ways (Robinson, 1991; Gorell Barnes *et al.*, 1995). Research indicates that the different ways have different sequelae and different outcomes. There is always a danger in extrapolating from trends in post-divorce and step-family literature to any single family.

In considering step-families, three areas of difference from biological families may be useful to note. Firstly, the formation of an intimate bond between adults in remarriage does not necessarily correlate with the establishment of intimate bonds between parents and step-children. New partners may be seen by children more as rivals for affection than as potential resources for themselves. Secondly, the relationship with former marriage partners and the way access arrangements fit with current relationships in the family need to be considered. The way in which a former partner, now a visiting partner, views a current step-parent will also have an impact on the way the child views a step-parent. Thirdly, general distinctions have been made in the research literature between biological parenting and social parenting. The concept of step-fathers becoming social parents to their step-children and moving away from their own biological children has been much discussed (Furstenberg, 1988; Kruk, 1992). The impact of such withdrawal of fathers from biological children and the effect of this on the children has not yet been documented.

In reviewing factors that contribute to adversity in childhood, the interaction between external social factors and intimate family relationships should always be considered. The way in which stressful life events amplify disadvantage or diminish resilience is also important to assess on an individual and family basis. Equally, factors that may be protective for some or all of the relationships in the family need recognition and acknowledgement by those who work with them. Issues of gender identity, and the way in which connections in the family are maintained or constrained for men and women within the family network, may also be important to consider in relation to the persistent use of drugs as a form of exchange or self-maintenance for young people (Dale and Emerson, 1994).

References

Boh K., Bak M., Clason C. *et al.* (1989) *Changing Patterns of European Family Life: A Comparative Analysis of 14 European Countries.* London: Routledge.

Belsky, J. and Pensky, E. (1988) Development history, personality and family relationships: Toward an emergent family system.In: Hinde, R. A. and Stevenson-Hinde, J. (eds.) *Relationships within Families: Mutual Influences,* pp. 193–217. Oxford: Oxford Scientific Publications.

Bowlby, J. (1980 *Attachment and loss, vol. 3 Loss, Sadness and Depression.* Hardmondsworth, Middlesex: Penguin Books.

Bretherton, I. (1985) Attachment theory: retrospect and prospect. In: Bretherton, I. and Waters, E. (eds.) *Growing Points of Attachment Theory and Research.* Monographs of the Society for Research in Child Development, **50**, (1–2).

Brown, G. (1990) Some public health aspects of depression. In: Goldberg, D. and Tantam, D. (eds.) *The Public Health Impact of Mental Disorder,* pp. 59–72.Toronto: Hogrefe and Huber.

Brown, G. (1991) *Life Events and Clinical Depression.* Practical Reviews in Psychiatry Series 3, No. 2. Education in Practice, Medical Tribune UK Ltd.

Brown, G. W., Harris, T. O. and Bifulco, A. (1986) Long term effects of early loss of a parent. In: Rutter, M., Izard, C. E. and Read, P. B. (eds.) *Depression in Young People: Developmental and Clinical Perspectives,* pp. 251–96. New York: Guilford Press.

Caspi, A. and Elder, G. H. (1988) Emergent family patterns: The intergenerational construction of problem behaviour and relationships. In: Hinde, R. A. and Stevenson-Hinde, J. (eds.) *Relationships within Families: Mutual Influences,* pp. 218–40.

Cook, J. and Watt, S. (1987) Racism, women and poverty. In: Glendinning, C. and Millar, J. (eds.) *Women and Poverty in Britain,* pp. 53–70. Brighton: Wheatsheaf Books, Harvester Press.

Cooklin, A. and Gorell Barnes, G. (1993) Taboos and social order: New encounters for family and therapist. In: Imber Black, E. (ed.) *Secrets in Families and Family Therapy,* London and New York: W. W. Norton & Co.

Cummings, E. M. (1987) Coping with background anger in early childhood. *Child Development,* **58**, 976–84.

Dale, B. and Emerson, P. (1994) The importance of being connected: implications for work with women addicted to drugs. In: Burck, C. and Speed, B. (eds.) *Gender Power and Relationships*, pp. 168–84. London: Routledge.

Dohrenwend, B. S. and Dohrenwend, B. P. (eds.) (1984) *Stressful Life Events and Their Contexts*. New Brunswick, NJ: Rutgers University Press.

Downey, G. and Coyne,J. C. (1990) Children of depressed parents: an integrative review. *Psychological Bulletin*, **108**, 50–76.

Elliott, J. and Richards, M. (1991) *Educational Performance and Behaviour, Before and After Parental Separation*. Child Care and Development Group; Free School Lane, Cambridge.

Emde, R. N. (1988) The effect of relationships on relationships: developmental approach to clinical intervention. In: Hinde, R. A. and Stevenson-Hinde, J. (eds.) *Relationships with Families: Mutual Influences*. Oxford: Scientific Publications.

Emery, R. E. (1989) Family violence. *American Psychologist*, **44**, 321–8.

Fernando, S. (1991) *Mental Health, Race and Culture*. Basingstoke and London: Mind Publications, MacMillan.

Furstenberg, F. F. (1988) Child care after divorce and remarriage. In; Hetherington, E. M. and Arasteh, J. D. (eds.) *Impact of Divorce, Single Parenting and Step-parenting on Children*, pp. 245–62. Hillsdale, New Jersey: Erlbaum.

Garmezy, N. (1985) Stress-resistant children: the search for protective factors. *Journal of Child Psychology and Psychiatry*, **4** (suppl.), 213–33.

Garmezy, N. (1987) Stress, competence and development: continuities in the study of schizophrenic adults, children vulnerable to psychopathology, and the search for stress-resistant children. *American Journal of Orthopsychiatry*, **57**, 159–74.

Garmezy, N. and Masten, A. (1994) Chronic Adversities. In: Rutter, M., Hersov, L. and Taylor, E. (eds.) *Child and Adolescent Psychiatry* (3rd ed.), pp. 191–208. Oxford: Blackwell Scientific Publications.

Glendinning, C. and Millar, J. (eds.) (1987) *Women and Poverty in Britain*. Brighton: Wheatsheaf Books.

Gorell Barnes, G. (1991*a*) Stepfamilies in context: the post divorce process. *Association for Child Psychology and Psychiatry Newsletter*, November, pp. 3–12.

Gorell Barnes, G. (1991*b*) Ambiguities in post divorce relationships. *Journal of Social Work Practice*, **5**, 143–50.

Gorell Barnes, G. (1995) Gender. In: Upton, G. and Davies, R. (eds.) *The Voice of the Child: A Handbook* (in press).

Gorell Barnes, G. and Cooklin, A. (1994) Family Therapy. In: Pokorney, M. and Clarkson, P. (eds.) *Handbook of Psychotherapy*, pp. 231–48. London: Routledge.

Gorell Barnes, G., Thompson, P., Daniel, G. and Burchhardt, N. (1995) *Growing up in step-families: life story interviews*. NCPS Cohort 1958. University of Essex, Department of Sociology and Institute of Family Therapy, London.

Guidobaldi, S. and Cleminshaw, H. (1985) Divorce, family health and child adjustment. *Family Relations*, **34**, 35–51.

Hardy, K. (1994) Deconstructing Race in Family Therapy. *Journal of Feminist Family Therapy* **5**, 5–33.

Harris T., Brown, G. W. and Bifulco, A. (1990) Loss of parent in childhood and adult psychiatric disorder: A tentative overall model. *Development and Psychopathology*, **2**, 311–28.

Henwood, M., Rimmer, L. and Wicks, M. (1987) *Inside the Family: Changing Roles of Men and Women*. Family Policy Studies Centre, Occasional Paper 6.

Hetherington, E. M. (1989) Coping with family transitions: winners, losers, and survivors. *Child Development*, **60**, 1–14.

Jenkins, J. M. and Smith, M. A. (1990) Factors protecting children living in disharmonious homes: maternal reports. *Journal of the American Academy of Child and Adolescent Psychiatry*, **29**, 60–9.

Kiernan, K. and Wicks, M. (1990) *Family Change and Future Policy*. Family Policy Studies Centre. Joseph Rowntree Memorial Trust.

Kolvin, I., Miller, F. J. W., Fleeting, M. and Kolvin, P. A. (1988*a*) Risk/ protective factors for offending with particular reference to deprivation. In: Rutter, M. (ed.) *Studies of Psychosocial Risk: The Power of Longitudinal Data*, pp. 77–95. Cambridge: Cambridge University Press.

Kolvin, I., Miller, F. J. W., Scott, D. McL., Gatznis, S. R. M. and Fleeting, M. (1988*b*) *Adversity and Destiny: Explorations in the Transmission of Deprivation - Newcastle Thousand Families Study*. Aldershot: Gower.

Kolvin, I., Miller, F. J. W., Fleeting, M. and Kolvin, P. A. (1988*c*) Social and parenting factors affecting criminal offence rates (findings from the Newcastle Thousand Families Study, 1947–1980). *British Journal of Psychiatry*, **152**, 80–90.

Kruk, E. (1992) Psychological and structural factors contributing to the disengagement of non-custodial fathers after divorce. *Family and Conciliation Court Review*, **30**, 81–101.

Lund, M. (1987) The non custodial father: common challenges in parenting after divorce. In: O'Brien, M. (ed.) *Reassessing Fatherhood: New Observations on Fathers of the Modern Family*. London: Sage.

Maccoby, E. E. (1980) *Social Development, Psychological Growth and the Parent–Child Relationship*. New York: Harcourt, Brace, Jovanovich.

Maine, M., Kaman, N. and Cassidy, J. (1985) Security in infancy, childhood and adulthood. A move to the level of representation. In: Bretherton, I. and Waters, E. (eds.) *Growing Points in Attachment Theory and Research*. Monographs of the Society in Research in Child Development, **50**, 1–2.

Masten, A. S., Best, K. M. and Garmezy, N. (1990) Resilience and development: contributions from the study of children who overcome adversity. *Development and Psychopathology*, **2**, 425–44.

Mills, M., Puckering, C., Pound, A. and Cox, A. (1984) What is it about depressed mothers that influences their children's functioning? In: Stephenson, J. E. (ed.) Recent Research in Developmental Psychopathology. *Journal of Child Psychology and Psychiatry*, Suppl. no. 4.

Mitchell, A. (1985) *Children in the Middle: Living Through Divorce*. London: Tavistock.

Quinton, D. and Rutter, M. (1984) Parents with children in care: 1. Current circumstances and parents. *Journal of Child Psychology and Psychiatry*, **25**, 211–31.

Patterson, G. R. and Capaldi, D. M. (1990) A mediational model for boys' depressive moods. In: Rolf, J., Masten, A. S., Cicchetti, D., Neuchterlein, K. H. and Weintraub, S. (eds.) *Risk and Protective Factors in the*

Development of Psychopathology, pp. 141–63. Cambridge: Cambridge University Press.

Radke-Yarrow, M. and Sherman, T. (1990) Hard growing: Children who survive. In: Rolf, J. E., Masten, A., Cicchetti, D., Neuchterlein, K. and Weintraub, S. (eds.) *Risk and Protective Factors in the Development of Psychopathology*, pp. 97–119. Cambridge: Cambridge University Press.

Robinson, M. (1991) *Family Transformation Through Divorce and Remarriage: A Systemic Approach*. London and New York: Tavistock/Routledge.

Rutter, M. (1978) Family, area and school influences in the genesis of conduct disorders. In: Hersov, L. A., Berger, M. and Schaffer, D. (eds.) *Aggression and Anti-Social Behavior in Childhood and Adolescence*, pp. 95–113. Oxford: Pergamon Press.

Rutter, M. (1979) Protective factors in children's responses to stress and disadvantage. In: Kent, M. W. and Rolf, J. E. (eds.) *Primary Prevention in Psychopathology: Social Competence in Children*, vol. 3, pp. 49–74. Hanover, NH: University Press of New England.

Rutter, M. (1984) Psychopathology and development. I. Childhood antecedents of adult psychiatric disorder. *Australian and New Zealand Journal of Psychiatry*, **18**, 225–34.

Rutter, M. (1985) Resilience in the face of adversity: Protective factors and resistance to psychiatric disorder. *British Journal of Psychiatry*, **147**, 598–611.

Rutter, M. (1987) Psychosocial resilience and protective mechanisms. *American Journal of Orthopsychiatry*, **57**, 316–31.

Rutter, M. (1990) Psychosocial resilience and protective mechanisms. In: Rolf, J., Masten, A. S., Cicchetti, D., Nuechterlein, K. H. and Weintraub, S. (eds.) *Risk and Protective Factors in the Development of Psychopathology*, pp. 181–214. Cambridge: Cambridge University Press.

Sameroff, A. J. and Seifer,R. (1990) Early contributors to developmental risk. In: Rolf, J. Masten, A. S., Cicchetti, D., Neuchterlein, K. H. and Weintraub, S (eds.) *Risk and Protective Factors in the Development of Psychopathology*. Cambridge: Cambridge University Press.

Sroufe, L. A. and Fleeson, J. (1988) The coherence of family relationships. In: Hinde, R. A. and Stevenson-Hinde, J. (eds.) *Relationships Within Families: Mutual Influence*, pp. 27–47. Oxford: Oxford Scientific Publications.

Stone, E. (1988) *Black Sheep and Kissing Cousins: How Our Family Stories Shape Us*. New York: Random House.

Zazlow, M. (1988*a*) Sex differences in children's response to parental divorce: research methodology and post divorce family focus. *American Journal of Orthopsychiatry*, **58**, 355–77.

Zazlow, M. (1988*b*). Sex differences in children's response to parental divorce: samples, variables, ages and sources. *American Journal of Orthopsychiatry*, **59**, 117–41.

4

Therapy in the eye of history: three episodes from the nineteenth century experience

GRIFFITH EDWARDS

Introduction

This book is about today's treatment of substance problems, and how, as of the minute, the generality of psychotherapeutic skills are to feed specialist activities. In this chapter we will stand back from imminent demands and examine how three episodes from nineteenth century history can speak to late twentieth century concerns. Rather as at a clinical conference, we will offer three cases for debate, but here our cases are not patients but the treatments given them.

Our first such presentation focuses on Thomas Trotter, a physician of the European Enlightenment, and what his book of 1804 may have to say about individual therapeutic processes. Next we turn to the Washingtonian movement of the 1840s, as exemplar of a non-professional and mutual help dimension in the treatment endeavour. Lastly and as our third example, we will examine developments in the last century in institutional treatment for substance problems – asylums, reformatories, and so on. The purpose is not to flatter ourselves by seeing past efforts as quaint, naive, or mistaken, nor that of drawing easy 'lessons from history'. The proper and far more difficult business is to discern processes, continuities, break points and basic issues, and where we stand in the long view of history. As with most usefully stimulating case conferences, one may hope that people leave the room still talking, rather than their being narcotised by easy answers.

Case 1. Thomas Trotter and inebriety as a habit to be broken

At the end of the eighteenth and beginning of the nineteenth century, the idea that inebriety might be a disease rather than a sin had become commonplace among leading physicians (Porter, 1985). That concept legitimised a medical role in response to excessive drinking (Levine, 1978; Edwards, 1992). Getting drunk was no longer merely a sin to be preached against and abhorred. Thomas Trotter was an Edinburgh-trained physician (Porter, 1988), who published his *Essay on Drunkenness* in 1804. With admitted arbitrariness we can take that volume (Trotter, 1804) as the starting point in the modern history of the psychotherapy of substance dependence.

Trotter asserted that 'The disease of inebriety is a habit of the mind'. He used the word 'habit' in a specific sense deriving from associationist psychology (itself later a source of Freudian psychoanalysis). The purpose of treatment was to break the habit and this would be done by distraction, setting up alternative activities, cajolery and persuasion. One is in the presence of an experienced, intuitive, and humane physician who was deploying an amalgam of interventions that would fit well with a modern cognitive behavioural approach. Quoted below are some excerpts from Trotter's text which illustrate his methods. Firstly, here is Trotter setting up the idea of habit as radical alternative to drunkenness as sin.

The priesthood hath poured forth its anathemas from the pulpit; and the moralist, no less severe, hath declaimed against it as a vice degrading to our nature. Both have meant well ... But the physical influence of custom, confirmed into habit, interwoven with the actions of our sentient system, and reacting on our mental part, have been entirely forgotten.

The next passage shows Trotter emphasising the need to make connections between cure and understanding of cause. He is in effect proposing that the physician should in every instance carry out a behavioural analysis.

The perfect knowledge of those remote causes which first induced the propensity to vinous liquors, whether they sprung from situation in life, or depended on any peculiar temperament of body, is necessary for conducting the cure.

The patient was seen as caught in a motivational dilemma, and the therapist would need to work on this conflict 'with patience and address'. By implication, listening and talking were the vital components of treatment:

The patient already knows, as well as the priest and moralist, that the indulgence is pernicious, and ultimately fatal ... but it is not so easy to convince him that you possess a charm that can recompense his feelings for the want of a grateful stimulus, or bestow on his nervous system sensations equally soothing and agreeable as he has been accustomed to receive from the bewitching spirit.

Trotter went on to emphasise the importance of the doctor–patient relationship:

The great point to be obtained is the confidence of the sick man; but this is not to be accomplished at a first visit ... When the physician has once gained the full confidence of his patient, he will find little difficulty in beginning his plan of cure. I have on several occasions wrought myself so much into the good graces of them, that nothing gave them so much alarm or uneasiness as the dread of declining my visits after they had been argued out of the pernicious practice.

Finally, much of Trotter's therapeutic technique can be seen as exemplified in the following passage:

. . . the necessity of studying the patient's temper and character, that we may acquire his confidence. These will lead us to the particular cause, time, and place of his love of the bottle. The danger of his continuing his career may be then calmly argued with him, and something proposed that will effectively wean his affections from it, and strenuously engage his attention. This must be varied according to circumstances, and must be left to the discretion of the physician.

So much for a note on the first of our case histories. Trotter may be read with profit by anyone practising today in this field as a source of startlingly fresh clinical wisdom, but for the historian the interest is likely to lie particularly in how his ideas on the treatment of inebriety derive from and reflect the beliefs of the eighteenth century Euopean enlightenment. Trotter's model of understanding fed through directly to his model of intervention. Furthermore, he may serve to persuade us that however fashions in therapy change, there are some insights that transcend time.

Case 2. The Washingtonians: a mutual help organisation of the 1840s

The next case study focuses on a mutual help movement that came into being in Baltimore in 1840 and which over the next few years flourished mightily, then to move equally quickly to decay and dissolution. The poignancy of this story resides in the sense of heady success with the reclamation of drunkards on a heroic scale never before seen, followed after just a few years by the movement's fading away. The context for this extraordinary development was the much wider American Temperance Movement (Wooley and Johnson, 1903; Sinclair, 1962; Gusfield, 1966), but the Washingtonians stood out as an organisation in large measure dedicated to helping the individual troubled drinker rather than just the carrying of a temperance or prohibition message to the population as a whole. We choose this as one of our three case studies so as to enter a reminder that a strong and important element of therapeutic activity in this field relates not to what professionals do in the name of treatment, but to the activities of self-help or mutual help groups, and many kinds of extra-professional and community-based activity.

The Washingtonian movement has attracted a substantial literature. This chapter will rely on material drawn from Temperance writers and also on later scholarly analysis. A particular debt is owed to Maxwell (1950) who traced important primary material, and to Blumberg (1980) who provides similarly rich sources in relation to Washingtonian activities at a local level in Paterson and Newark, New Jersey.

Baltimore, a night in April 1840

On a Thursday evening in April 1840, six heavy-drinking friends were spending a convivial evening in a tavern. They comprised a tailor, a carpenter, a coach maker, two blacksmiths and a silversmith. Seemingly more as a joke than with any serious intent, four of these men moved off to hear a public lecture that was being given in the city by a visiting temperance advocate. When the group got together again the idea crystallised that all of them should renounce drink, sign a pledge, and set up their own Temperance Society – 'the idea seemed to take wonderfully; and the more they laughed and talked over it, the more they were pleased with it' (Harrison, 1860, quoted by Maxwell, 1950). By Sunday the new society was up and running with its officers elected. A form of pledge had been drafted and ascribed in the following terms:

We, whose names are annexed, desirous of forming a society for our mutual benefit and to guard against a pernicious practice which is injurious to our health, standing, and families, do pledge ourselves as gentlemen that we will not drink any spirituous or malt liquors, wine or cider.

Thus was founded an association dedicated to 'mutual support', and on the evident premise that the group was more likely to achieve and maintain sobriety than isolated, individual effort. These men had drunk together, and now they would be sober together. Unlike some other temperance affiliates, they would give up all types of alcohol and not just spirits. They named their association the 'Washington Temperance Society' in honour of George Washington. At first the group continued to hold its meetings in their usual tavern, but before long there were complaints from the tavern keeper that his best customers were being taken away from him. The society moved off to meet in someone's home, and before long a hall had to be hired to accommodate growing numbers.

Statistics of success

The Temperance movement as a whole often attempted to win hearts and minds by quoting gigantic figures for success and conversion, but without too scrupulous attention to audit. The first anniversary parade of the Washingtonians was able to muster 'about 1000 reformed drunkards and 5000 members and friends' (Maxwell, 1950), and the movement was by then spreading to other US cities. Huge numbers of people were signing the pledge – a tour through New York, New Jersey and Pennsylvania allegedly brought over 23 000 new signatures. In 1842 10 000 signatures were won in Illinois, 30 000 in Kentucky and a massive 60 000 in Ohio. The movement was expanding exponentially and one estimate would suggest that by 1843 about four million Americans had signed the Washingtonian pledge. As for the proportion of the total who were dependent drinkers or experiencing a serious drink problem, the figures are again very unreliable. As Maxwell noted, one is up against the problem of interpreting the meaning of counts conducted within such categories as 'hard drinkers often drunken', 'confirmed drinkers', 'sot', and all the way through to 'tipplers in a fair way to becoming sots'.

Methods of working
Local responsibility

Working with a common pledge and guidelines for articles of association, there appears to have been considerable responsibility left to local associations: officers were elected and a small membership fee levied. The taking of the pledge was tantamount to becoming a member. The association embraced those who had experienced a problem, but also moderate drinkers who wanted to become teetotal for reasons of personal choice. A Washingtonian association might be a new foundation or it could develop out of an existing temperance meeting of a more generic kind. The majority of members were men, but women also were admitted.

What happened at association meetings

Weekly meetings would be held in a public hall. A widely quoted precept enjoined members both to attend and recruit – 'Let every man be present, and himself bring a man'. A hymn would be sung or a prayer said, and then a 'reformed drunkard' would tell the story of his degradation, despair and reclamation. The Washingtonians seem very soon to have realised the power and engagement of this kind of personal statement. Others would get up and make further contributions and there would then be the ritual of pledge signing.

Public meetings

Besides the more routine kind of meeting described above, the Washingtonians also held large public meetings of a more revivalist or missionary kind, especially as they moved into new geographical territory. Parades and torchlight processions might then be part of the show (Sinclair, 1962). Daniels (1878) described the common features of the kind of address that was likely to be given at such meetings:

Personal experiences, droll stories and sharp jokes at the expense of drunkards and drunkard-makers; imitations of the antics and fooleries of men under the influence of liquor; sharp thrusts at the avariciousness and meanness of the liquor sellers and at the tricks of liquor makers, formed the staple of the lecturing under the Washingtonian movement.

Certain individuals achieved fame as platform orators – 'Who of our older citizens has not listened to the thrilling and simple experience of John Hawkins as he portrayed the misery of the drunkard and told the touching story of his little daughter, Hannah, persuading him to reform?' (Gough, 1881). Washingtonians meetings were often the best show in town.

Therapeutic processes

The local weekly meetings could be where the drinker found the gateway to the help he needed. That help came partly through the giving of hope and the simple assurance that he was capable of 'reform'. The role model provided by recovered drinkers must have been an essential ingredient. There was the immediate sense of welcome, and the Washingtonian ethic put much emphasis on love and succour as opposed to harshness or denunciation. Here is an extract from an address given by John Hawkins, which shows 'the tone and spirit of that brotherly work' (Daniels, 1878):

Drunkard! come up here, you can reform . . . We don't slight the drunkard; we love him, we nurse him, as a mother does her infant learning to walk.

I tell you, be kind to those men; they have peculiar feelings when the boys run after them and hoot at them.

On another occasion Hawkins is quoted as saying 'I'll never slight a drunkard as long as I live: he needs sympathy and is worth of it. Poor and miserable as he is, he did not design to have become a drunkard, and people have too long told him he cannot reform. But now we assure him he can reform, and we show ourselves . . . as evidence of that fact'. (Daniels, 1878).

Outreach work

Besides psychological assistance to the process of recovery that the Washingtonians offered to the troubled drinkers who came their way, these associations were willing to go out and look for recruits, and would offer help of a practical kind. Food, shelter and clothing might be made available. Newly sober men would be boarded out in the homes of Washingtonian families. A variety of club houses, day shelters and lodging houses were opened, and a house in Boston achieved particular fame as a fully developed insitution (see p.68 below). This outreach work was helped by the activity of Martha Washington Associations, a kind of women's auxiliary which came into existence in many localities. These groups worked partly through raising funds and dispensing material help to newly recovering men, but at least some of them took on a special responsibility for helping women who had drinking problems.

Why the Washingtonian movement failed

A variety of explanations for the demise of this movement were put forward by contemporary or near-contemporary commentators. One such explanation was offered by Gough (1881) in terms of an inability to handle the religious connection successfully, with clergymen feeling that they were being elbowed off the platform by reformed drunkards:

Men became leading reformers who were not qualified by experience, or training, or education, to lead, and out of them a class sprung up who became dictatorial, and sometimes insolent. Irreligious men insulted in some instances ministers of religion who had been hard workers for temperance; reformed drunkards sneered at those who had never been intemperate, as if former degradation was the only qualification for leadership.

Further destructive influences may have included the development of faction fighting between the Washingtonians and other temperance groups with whom they had at the start co-operated rather well, unwise involvement in local politics, the scandal that would follow the 'backsliding' into drink of a prominent and far from anonymous lecturer, and the public's sense of satiation or ennui, as it was before long more battered than thrilled by yet another story of hideous degradation and miraculous recovery.

The enormous complexity of Temperance history should be acknowledged (Harrison, 1971), and the pace and force of contextual events. Blumberg (1980) has argued that the Washingtonians were in effect overtaken by the historical movement that was beginning to give a more dominant influence to the elements of Temperance that were looking for political solutions and beginning to lean towards prohibition. The Washingtonians were individual-oriented, and Temperance was moving toward an increasingly social orientation. Whatever the interacting influences, local and immediate or related to the larger groundswell, within a few years a movement that had attracted Abraham Lincoln to one of its meetings, packed the public halls, spread like fire across a continent, helped troubled drinkers to recovery in huge numbers, explored the power of group processes and of the recovered individual as role model, and combined an ethic of compassion with material help, had become a shadowy and to some a rather embarrassing event of the past. That is not to deny the continuing influences of the Washingtonians on the evolving Temperance story – the memory trace was not wiped out.

What does the Washingtonian movement tell us about therapy?

The temptingly facile approach to interpretation of this story would be to view the Washingtonians as primitive precursor to Alcoholics Anonymous (AA), make point-by-point comparisons of an obvious kind, and offer a set of conclusions that congratulate AA on its organisational acumen while identifying aspects of the earlier movement's organisational ineptness. A more cautious and valid approach to analysis of such social movements must emphasise the extraordinary embeddedness of these phenomena in the political and social contexts of their times. A 'compare and contrast' approach to the Washingtonians and AA might if carefully handled be in some way productive, but the handling would have to be historically sensitive.

Let's, however, turn from the fascinating but difficult questions that attach to the Washingtonians as social movement, and focus on the more strictly therapeutic aspects of the story. As stated earlier, the justification for including this phenomenon as one of our case presentations lies in its forceful reminder that therapy is not something uniquely done by professionals. Around the contention this early instance of a mutual help movement would then seem to cluster a number of still pertinent questions:

1. *What are the special therapeutic powers and qualities that the 'recovered person' brings to therapeutic contacts?* We have referred already to the probable power of role modelling, and the Washingtonians also illustrate the ability of the recovering drinker to express love and compassion in a way that might seem cloying, possessive and unhealthy to the professional.

2. *How can other sectors and recovering individuals work together?* The latter days of the Washingtonian movement showed clashes between 'reformed drunkards' who were accused of being 'insolent' or 'dictatorial', and the clergy. Those tensions parallel boundary disputes between 'recovered addicts' and treatment professionals. If there is to be a productive partnership, questions will have to be repeatedly resolved in different generations and circumstances relating to status and ownership, as well as working methods.

3. *Waiting for the patients to come or chasing after them.* The Washingtonians were willing to go out and search the streets for drinkers whom they would rescue. The medical tradition has been to wait for the patient to make an appointment or join the waiting-list, although a developing emphasis on outreach challenges that position. AA has never proselytised or gone out to rescue.

4. *Mixing therapy with food, blankets and shelter.* The contrast between AA's refusal ever to become involved in good works and the Washingtonian provision of practical support is again acute. As regards hospital practice, most professional therapists would probably view it as anti-therapeutic to offer a client so much as the price of a meal, although a referral to the social work department might deal with those practical problems that were so much part of the Washingtonian enterprise. Voluntary agencies have traditionally been more willing to cross this kind of boundary, as witnessed for instance by the Salvation Army. The large and underlying question is how far psychological treatment and material help are at any deep

level conceptually and operationally distinct, or whether the Washingtonians were boldly ahead of their time in seeing a unity. The modern concept of 'community reinforcement' revisits this question (Azrin *et al.*, 1982).

So much for some of the questions that were flagged by 1840, Baltimore, and what followed. We are not offering a framed temperance text, but material for debate.

Case 3. The rise of institutional treatment

For our third case story, let's take as starting point *The Disease of Inebriety*, a book published in 1893 under the auspices of the American Association for the Study and Cure of Inebriety, but probably written by T. D. Crothers (Crothers, 1893). Set out in the Introduction were the principles and purposes of the American Association for the Study and Cure of Inebriety, a society that had been founded in 1870, in New York City (Blumberg, 1978). With minor abbreviation these articles read as follows:

1. Inebriety is a disease.
2. It is curable as other diseases are.
3. The constitutional tendency to this disease may be either inherited or acquired: but the disease is often induced by the habitual use of alcohol or other narcotic substance.
4. Alcohol . . . as a medicine . . . should be prescribed with great caution.
5. All methods hitherto employed for the treatment of inebriety that have not recognised the disordered physical condition caused by alcohol, opium or other narcotics, have proved inadequate in its cure: hence the establishment of *hospitals* for the special treatment of inebriety . . . becomes a positive need of the age.
6. . . . this Association urges that every large city should have its local and temporary hospital for both the reception and care of inebriates: and that every State should have hospitals for their permanent detention and treatment . . .
7. Finally, the officers of such hospitals and asylums should have ample legal power of control over their patients, and authority to retain them a sufficient length of time for their permanent cure.

In chronicling the history of the institutional treatment movement, Crothers himself identified two landmark events. First, there was the opening in 1845 of the Washingtonian Hall in Boston, Massachussets, a small refuge that provided shelter and a sober environment for drinkers who were trying to break with their alcohol dependence. The second institution to which Crothers referred was for him and the Association not so much a landmark as an icon. This was the Binghampton Hospital, opened in 1864, and otherwise known as the New York State Inebriates Asylum (Ryfins, 1949).

Binghampton was the brainchild of a physician from Maine, Dr J. Edward Turner. It had its precursors and successors, and the extensive history which Braumohl (1990) has given of inebriate institutions in Canada and the United States over the years 1840 to 1920, puts in due perspective this one manifestation of widely varied types of institutional developments that catered for different kinds of problem. For eight years Turner worked to raise the necessary funds for Binghampton and secure the needed legislative backing from the State. According to Crothers it was 'the first institution of the kind ever organised'. The hospital kept its doors open for 14 years, during which time it treated 2 344 inmates, but for much of this period it was beset by acrimonious controversy. Binghampton was finally turned into an 'insane asylum' and 'Turner shared the fate of all reformers and benefactors of the world, in the obloquy and disgrace of being driven away from the creation of his own genius' (Crothers, 1893).

Crother's *Disease of Inebriety* gave an update on the American institutional situation in 1893. Some 15 years after the closure of Binghampton, Crothers claimed that a dozen hospitals were carrying on similar work in the United States. He also stated that the institutional movement had at that period become well established internationally:

In Europe, over sixty hospitals for the physical care and treatment of inebriates are in active operation today. There are two in Australia, one in China, two in India, one in Ceylon, three in Africa, and one in Mexico. While these institutions vary widely in plan and methods, the central idea is the physical treatment of the inebriate and his malady.

And it was in large measure the emphasis on physical treatment of inebriety conceived as essentially a physical disease (an exhaustion of nerve cells), which characterised the nineteenth century institutional approach to the treatment of alcohol dependence. Rest and rehabilitation, a healthy diet, faradic stimulation and Turkish baths were essential ingredients in this approach. Crothers even saw a place in his armentarium for leeches:

> If inebriety is associated with suicidal tendencies it will be important to ascertain whether any cerebral congestion exists, and if so a few leeches applied to the head, followed by an active cathartic, will relieve the local irritation. In the absence of any positive active cerebral symptom, the prolonged warm bath and the continued exhibition of morphine will be the best treatment until the suicidal idea disappears.

This emphasis on the physical elements in treatment deserves note, but that there were elements of milieu therapy and moral exhortation should also be recognised. Essentially what was being brought over during these decades to the treatment of inebriety was the mix of methods that characterised the contemporary asylum movement in general, with its favouring of compulsion, the quiet retreat, a long stay, an ordered regime, physical treatments, and moral improvement. The psychological element within such programmes was, though, much impoverished in comparison to Trotter's insights and practice. Here, for instance, is a passage in which Crothers (1893) described his view as to what the psychological element in institutional treatment might be expected to achieve.

> Such results [sobriety] may not be reached by the final and total extinction of the morbid desire for alcohol, so much as by a development and cultivation of opposite and ennobling qualities, which by their vital action, hold the depraved mental tendencies of the subject in constant and absolute subjection, so that they become as inoperative as if they did not exist.

A brilliantly revealing statement delineating the mix of approaches which should provide the lineaments of the medico-moral regime in any well-run inebriates' home was given by Norman Kerr (1889), one of Crothers's English contemporaries and a key figure in British campaigns for legally backed institutional treatment of the inebriate (Berridge, 1990). Kerr wrote:

> There is this benefit in such a life under one roof ... In well-managed Homes there are discussions which stimulate thought, social gatherings which promote good fellowship, musical evenings, productive of real pleasure, sacred concerts and services which purify the heart and strengthen the moral control. Most of the patients felt constrained by the general tone of the community in a good Home ... a tendency to infuse into all a determination to perform the duties which every member of a well organised family circle always owes to every other member of it ... There will be innocent amusement and healthful recreation in abundance, with facilities for scientific study, for the exercise of handicraft, and for artistic work.

Kerr went on:

There will be adequate medical supervision ... The patient will be under moral as well as hygienic and medical treatment. Valuable as is the assistance from certain therapeutic agents in the arresting of the disease ... of the aid from *Materia Medica* moral treatment is the compliment. The latter is as essential as the former. The concentration of the patient's thoughts upon himself, his obliquity to truth (an obliquity at once physical and moral), are most effectually redirected by the unconscious force of a masterful friend. Personal contact with the medical guide and controlling spirit, as well as with his fellow patients, will do more to draw the narcomania out of his morbid egotism than a hundred lectures or a thousand seminars.

The expansion of institutional provisions with an edge of compulsion was over the latter part of the nineteenth century a dominant, campaigning issue on both sides of the Atlantic (Collins, 1903; Berridge, 1990).

Institutions for inebriates and today's concerns

How can a look back at the nineteenth century history of the inebriate institution (hospital, home, reformatory, call it by any name), throw light on our concern better to understand the genesis, nature and predicaments of our modern psychotherapies? Several themes could be brought into focus. First, if Trotter's and the institutional approach are compared, one is persuaded that the models of understanding employed by therapists or their age and times, are likely to be powerful determinants of the model of care that is deployed. Trotter believed that the problem was the habit and the habit had to be broken by psychological means. Crothers and his colleagues crudely neurologised inebriety as a physical disorder stemming from the exhaustion of brain cells; so for these practitioners the response had to be physical.

That analysis can, of course, immediately be seen as in some ways too simple. The institutionalists believed in the 'moral' element to treatment as well as medical. On occasion moral meant little other than moralistic or exhortatory, but with Kerr if not Crothers moral could also mean psychological in a wider sense – Kerr understood both the importance of the therapist and the influence of the milieu and the group. Perhaps what we need to note as a pertinent and continuing theme is that the question of how morality is to be handled when we are dealing with people who engage in disapproved behaviour, is never done. Crothers and Kerr tended to wear their moral position more openly than would today be fashionable, but that does not mean that our contemporary world has once and for all and successfully disposed of the moral dilemma.

Another theme that should be identified is the extent to which the background of general therapeutic practice is likely to influence the specialist practice with substance dependence. Trotter wrote with wonderful sensitivity on 'drunkenness', but he wrote as a physician who practised within the ideas and methods which were influencing medicine in his time. Institutional treatment of inebriety evolved as the almost guaranteed consequence of the asylum age.

Lastly and in relation to Binghampton, we can identify the grand theme of institutional entrepreneurship. We might guess that this is a theme that was, is, and will be a characteristic of the substance treatment business for all time. In the nineteenth century it was the Reformatory and its like that were being cloned and multiplied, with Crothers proudly notching up the international tally. The spread of that kind of institution no doubt resulted from many different processes. There was also an element of professional aggrandisement and a staking out of an arena for nascent specialism, and at times there was money to be made. The fact that institutions had been established in Australia, China, Ceylon, India, Africa and Mexico suggests that therapy could also be a vehicle for imperialism. To track and explain within context the latter-day international dissemination of AA, the Minnesota Model, methadone, relapse prevention, or the primary care approach, would provide a set of enthralling research questions.

Three case histories: no summing up

Throughout this chapter we have sought to emphasise that history is not a repository of moral tales. To sum up under a few neat headings the impact which each of us might variously derive from a reading of Trotter, reflection on the Washingtonian story, or on analysis of nineteenth century institutional entrepreneurship (and the application of leeches), would negate the proper impact of the whole experience. Continued cogitation rather than the comfort of bullet points must be the proper order of the day. We might, however, wish to plead that when reading the chapters that follow and that deal with complex contemporary issues, a little personal space should be allowed us for wonder and distance. We need to step outside our present world, look at it in historical perspective, and acknowledge that our present concerns are in many respects a matter of long continuities.

References

Azrin, N. H., Sisson, R. W., Meyers, R. and Godley, M. (1982) Alcoholism treatment by disulfiram and community reinforcement therapy. *Journal of Behaviour Therapy and Experimental Psychiatry*, **135**, 105–12.

Berridge, V. (1990) Special Issue. The Society for the Study of Addiction 1884–1988. *British Journal of Addiction*, **85**, 983–1087.

Blumberg, L. G. (1978) The American Association for the Study and Cure of Inebriety. *Alcoholism: Clinical and Experimental Research*, **2**, 234–40.

Blumberg, L. G. (1980) The significance of the alcohol Prohibitionists for the Washington Temperance Societies. With special reference to Paterson and Newark, New Jersey. *Journal of Studies on Alcohol*, **41**, 37–77.

Braumohl, J. (1990) Inebriate institutions in North America, 1840–1920. *British Journal of Addiction*, **85**, 1187–204.

Brown, E. M. (1985) 'What shall we do with the inebriate?' Asylum treatment and the disease concept of alcoholism in the nineteenth century. *Journal of the History of Behavioural Science*, **21**, 48–59.

Collins, W. J. (1903) An address on the institutional treatment of inebriety. *British Journal of Inebriety*, **1**, 97–115.

Crothers, T. D. (1893) *The Disease of Inebriety from Alcohol, Opium and other Narcotic Drugs, its Etiology, Pathology, Treatment and Medico-legal Relations.* Arranged and compiled by the American Association for the Study and Cure of Inebriety. Bristol: John Wright and Co.

Daniels, W. H. (1878) *The Temperance Reform and its Great Reformers: An Illustrated History.* New York: Nelson and Phillips.

Edwards, G. (1992) Problems and dependence: the history of two dimensions. In: Lader, M. and Edwards, G. (eds.) *The Nature of Alcohol and Drug Related Problems*, pp. 1–13. Society for the Study of Addiction Monograph No. 2. Oxford: Oxford University Press.

Gough, J. B. (1881) *Sunlight and Shadow or Gleanings from my Life Work.* Hartford, Conn: A. D. Worthington and Company.

Gusfield, J. R. (1966) *Symbolic Crusade: Status Policies and the American Temperance Movement.* Urbana Ill.: University of Illinois Press.

Harrison, D. (1860) *A Voice from the Washingtonian Home.* Boston: Redding and Co.

Harrison, B. (1971) *Drink and the Victorians: The Temperance Question in England.* London: Faber and Faber.

Kerr, N. (1889) *Inebriety, its Etiology, Pathology, Treatment and Jurisprudence,* 2nd edn. London: H. K. Lewis.

Levine, H. G. (1978) The disease of addiction: changing conceptions of habitual drunkenness in America. *Journal of Studies on Alcohol*, **39**, 143–44.

Maxwell, M. A. (1950) The Washingtonian Movement. *Quarterly Journal of Studies on Alcohol*, **11**, 411–51.

Porter, R. (1985) The drinking man's disease: the 'pre-history' of alcoholism in Georgian Britain. *British Journal of Addiction*, **80**, 385–96.

Porter, R. (1988) Introduction. In: Trotter, T. *An Essay, Medical Philosophical and Chemical, on Drunkenness and its Effects on the Human Body*, reprinted edn, pp. ix–x. London: Routledge.

Ryfins, S. (1949) Joseph Turner and the first inebriate asylum. *Quarterly Journal of Studies on Alcohol*, **10**, 127–34.

Sinclair, A. (1962) *Prohibition. The Era of Excess.* London: Faber and Faber.

Trotter, T. (1804) *An Essay, Medical, Philosophical and Chemical, on Drunkenness, and its Effects on the Human Body*. London: T. N. Longman and O. Rees.

Wooley, J. G. and Johnson, W. E. (1903) *Temperance Progress in the Century*. London: Linscott Publishing Company.

Part two
Treatments

5

Psychotherapy: why do some need more and some need less?

SUSAN DAVISON

Introduction

Psychoanalytic psychotherapy draws upon psychoanalysis for its theory and its technique, the main difference between the two being the frequency with which sessions are held. The former offers sessions one to three times and the latter four to five times per week. Both aim to understand, through the analysis of transference and resistance, the unconscious underpinning of symptoms and dysfunctional relationships. Psychoanalytic theory is still evolving, partly through dialogue among competing theoretical perspectives (Frosch, 1987), partly through the challenges thrown up by patients who are dificult to treat (Klein, 1932; Rosenfeld, 1965; Searles, 1965; Kernberg *et al.*, 1989) and partly in articulation with adjacent disciplines such as developmental psychology (Stern, 1985; Murray-Parkes *et al.*, 1991).

A parallel development has been various attempts to modify psychoanalytic technique in the service of brief dynamic therapies (Malan, 1963; Ryle, 1975, 1990; Davanloo, 1978; Luborsky, 1984; Strupp and Binder, 1984; Malan and Osimo, 1992; Sifneos, 1992). These have been shown to be useful where treatment trials have been done and to have roughly the same potency as cognitive therapy, in various clinical settings (Crits-Christoph, 1992).

In this chapter the focus will be on advances in clinical concepts in relation to change and the psychotherapeutic process, rather than the current state of process and outcome research in psychodynamic psychotherapy. There has been an enormous research effort in this area in the USA and, with the 'third generation' psychotherapy research projects, findings are beginning to emerge that have clinical relevance. Good recent surveys of the state of the field can be found by Dahl *et al.* (1988), Luborsky *et al.* (1988) and Luborsky and Crits-Christoph

(1990). These projects have built on the experience of the Menniger Foundation Psychotherapy Research Project (Kernberg *et al.*, 1972; Horowitz, 1974; Appelbaum, 1977; Wallerstein, 1986). We will be drawing here on a particular line of development within psychoanalysis that is peculiarly British, the Kleinian tradition (Spillius, 1983, 1988), and which contributes to our understanding of some of the psychodynamic forces that may drive a person to become addicted to alcohol or drugs. For reviews of the psychoanalytic literature on the addictions see Rosenfeld (1960, 1964), Yorke (1970), Meissner (1981) and Smaldino (1991).

There are undoubtedly patients who benefit from brief interventions, as will be shown below in the first two clinical examples, yet there are also those for whom longer-term psychoanalytic psychotherapy is their only hope for significant change, as in the second two examples. Following a description of these cases the discussion will turn to the differences between those people who are able to make use of the brief interventions and those for whom more time is an essential ingredient. The existence of a partner or a family able and willing to participate, probably does indicate a social ability that favours brief therapy. Whether working with families, couples or individuals, the theoretical model considered here is psychoanalytic. With families one may assume that significant transferences and projections are occurring between members of the family rather than to the therapist (Scharff, 1985; Slipp, 1988), so that in practice the technique employed with families and couples differs from that of the psychoanalytic session.

Four case studies

Case 1. Six sessions of marital therapy free a couple to find their own way forward

Mr and Mrs A. were offered six sessions of marital therapy when Mr A. presented with depression of fairly recent onset. He had found himself trapped in a situation of his own choosing that, to his distress, replicated in important respects the situation from which he had struggled to free himself during adolescence. He and his wife had met at university, and after a short, chaste courtship had married six years previously. They were members of an enthusiastic evangelical church, which occupied much of their free time. Recently they had adopted two toddlers as, sadly, they had discovered they were infertile.

Mr A.'s family had migrated to Britain from the Far East following the death of his father. He had many siblings whom his mother had brought up devotedly in difficult circumstances. He loved and respected his mother enormously, but had felt dreadfully constrained by her and the wider family's expectation that he adhere strictly to their cultural and religious customs. He had escaped to university in another town with relief, and later converted to Christianity. This and his marriage to a Caucasian girl caused his mother much grief, though she still wanted him to return to live nearby. Mrs A. was the only child of a lonely, depressed, demanding mother and a rather distant public-spirited father who was very busy outside the home. Mrs A. was afraid that she was becoming just like her mother and was in fact driving her husband to work longer and longer hours to avoid her.

Married life had proved rather a shock to both of them, and, having shared their difficulties with the church, they were the recipients of much prayerful concern and advice, not all of it helpful. Mr A. felt the church was endorsing his wife's sexual inhibition and self-sacrifice while disapproving of his wish for more fun. She had become all duty and he was fast becoming delinquent as, once again, he was up against the demands and expectations of a rigid religious system. An added pressure on him was his family's complaints that he was neglecting his filial duties.

Many things were discussed during the six marital therapy sessions, and in small ways many things improved, as Mr and Mrs A. began to be able to listen to one another again and to meet one another half way. A crucial issue turned out to be that Mr A. was a much more confident parent than his wife. She felt doubly unsupported because, without the inauguration of pregnancy, she missed out on the care and protection she felt other mothers would have had. She felt cruelly left out and upstaged when her husband romped with the children at bedtime. When he understood her need of cuddles too, she was much better able to be sympathetic to his dilemmas.

By the last session they happily reported that they were enjoying their marriage in all its aspects and indeed had resolved to adopt two more children when they were able. Six months later Mr A. wrote to say that he was feeling completely better.

Case 2. Chaos, one family meeting – and seven years later . . .

Miss B. had been offered a preliminary interview with her parents and two elder brothers. The referral had been to a therapeutic community for consideration of in-patient psychotherapy since local resources had been tried without success. Miss B. had, over the preceding 18 months, become so self-conscious that she refused to go to school. Instead she spent hours in front of the mirror adjusting her appearance, plucking her eyebrows, squeezing blackheads, cutting her hair, applying and taking off make-up. Regularly she would become so filled with frustration and despair that she sought to take her own life, ending up in hospital as a result. Her parents were at their wits' end. They had tried covering all the mirrors in the house and confiscating scissors and tweezers; they offered their daughter a personal taxi service, and when she passed her driving test, bought her a little car.

Both older siblings had left home and were doing well in good jobs. Miss B. was, by common consent, the brightest of the three and, before she became ill, was well set to enter university. At the family meeting Mrs B. was somewhat detached, exuding disapproval of the whole proceedings. She wondered whether we could recommend some suitable medication for her daughter. Mr B. was more overtly upset; he believed that if only his daughter could be prevailed upon to let her hair grow, all would be well. One of her brothers took the view that his little sister was 'spoilt rotten' and a little discipline would not come amiss. There was a general expectation that our more powerful therapy would succeed where their own efforts had failed.

The therapist was at pains to emphasise that while we might aim to help Miss B. to live with her imperfections, we would be no better at enforcing the strategies they had tried than they were, since Miss B. was obviously a very determined young woman. However, it was distressing to see her wasting her talents; was a long period in hospital preferable to going back to school?

Agitatedly, Mr B. insisted they could no longer cope. Only two days previously, Miss B. had rushed out of the house, jumped into her car and driven off. Just that morning, she had been threatening to kill herself, and he had given chase. They must have covered over 30 miles of narrow country roads at high speed. Miss B., who until this point had been silent and sullen, joined in the account, explaining contemptuously how easily she had given her father the slip and bought yet another pair of scissors. Both father and daughter became animated, smiling and laughing for the first time. Mother remained frosty. This exchange clarified that father and daughter were involved in an excited dance to which Miss B. called the tune. Father was signalling his wish to be released from it, yet his wife appeared unable to help. Further discussion clarified that Mrs B. had not thought there had been a serious risk of suicide, a point her husband readily conceded.

Mr and Mrs B. opted for a further family meeting, rather than insisting that their daughter be admitted to the therapeutic community. However, it was agreed that life had become intolerable for them, and that should there be another crisis before the next meeting, they would ask their local services for help. The following day, the therapist received a call from their GP. He had been called in to find the house in uproar. What should he do? He wanted to sedate Miss B., who was rampaging about the house threatening suicide. It was agreed that he should do so, framing it as a means of giving her parents a rest, for two or three days at the most. The next family meeting was cancelled by Mr B. A little later he wrote to say things had settled down. They had worked out a way for Miss B. to continue her studies and take her exams. She was calmer and happier, though still very self-conscious. She had acknowledged to her parents that her preoccupation with her appearance was abnormal, but had agreed not to let it dominate their lives.

A follow-up seven years later revealed that Miss B. had gone on to University and had nearly finished a post-graduate degree. She was living with her boyfriend, a fellow student, and Mr and Mrs B. commented that 'she had been just fine for the last three to four years now, which is a great load off our minds'.

Case 3. A tormented young woman, two years of twice-weekly psychotherapy, and eight years later . . .

Miss J. was 27 years old, single, unemployed and already had a long history of contact with various psychiatric services when she was assessed by a colleague. A previous attempt at out-patient psychotherapy had broken down and she had spent 18 months in a therapeutic community without discernible benefit. Later she had been offered a place at a Day Hospital, which though psychodynamically informed, was a place of last resort. She was described by the consultant there as 'quite the most tormented young woman to have been seen in a long time'.

Her appearance was extraordinary. She was festooned with bright scarves and beads so as to resemble a mad woman. Her communication was disconcertingly disconnected, though it was possible to follow a thread of meaning if one did not attend too closely to the lack of logic. Descriptively she suffered from a severe personality disorder with borderline and hysterical features (DSM-III-R). Her symptomatology was florid and diverse.

Her family background and childhood experience had been very difficult. Both her parents had been mentally ill, as well as her maternal grandmother. Much of the care of her young siblings and the home had devolved onto her, as her elder sister was disabled. Her parents parted when she was a teenager and she left home at 19, knowing then that she needed help. An unplanned pregnancy by a violent boyfriend and its termination precipitated a state of unredeemed hopelessness, cruelly tormenting guilt and suicidal impulses, with a wheedling voice encouraging her to kill herself in one of a number of violent ways. It terrified her as did the recurring conviction that she was being followed by an ill-intentioned man.

She also suffered from multiple phobias, the avoidance of which seriously restricted her life. She had used a number of street drugs, including LSD, and had difficulty controlling her drinking. Once intoxicated she became totally disinhibited, which could put her in danger. She lived alone because she could not tolerate the proximity of other people, yet she was intensely lonely. She marked the passing of the days by hoarding empty packets and tins; she kept a 'stash' of pills as insurance against the time she could not go on. Yet others perceived her as capable, efficient and reliable. They discounted her nightmare world as colourful exaggeration, and it is probable that the more she felt misunderstood, the more she had to emphasise her desperation. She found it a great relief that the therapist who had assessed her recognised the nature of her illness and yet did not pronounce her hopeless. During the intervening nine months while she waited for a vacancy, she began to venture out from her lonely and constricted routine, and to put her life in some order.

The details of the two years of twice-weekly psychotherapy cannot be recounted here. Suffice to say that it was a difficult and testing experience for both therapist and patient. It had the feel of a real life-and-death struggle in which the therapist was experienced as a number of dangerous, corrupt, or weak figures in the transference. Slowly, as many of her symptoms abated and she grew calmer, she became better able to take things in. For the first time in years she took up her studies and set about gaining the qualifications to go to university. The therapy ended prematurely when she had secured a place at a university some distance from the therapist. She had by then a small band of trusted friends and was taking her first tentative steps with a young male friend. At follow-up five years later she had successfully gained a degree and had started a job. At the time of writing she is looking for further help as she experienced a crisis that indicated that all was not well, but she is a very different person from the frightened, lonely woman of eight years ago.

Case 4. *Misery and anger, six years of individual psychotherapy and a happy outcome*

Miss K. was a thin young woman who always dressed in black as a dramatic personification of a 'streak of misery'. She specialised in alienating people. She had been depressed since the death of her grandmother 15 years earlier. She despised her father, who had divorced her mother not long after, for his weakness and cruelty. This contempt extended to her grandfather and other male members of the family who, according to her, mistreated women in order to enhance their pathetic self-importance. She was protectively attached to her mother who had suffered for years from agoraphobia. She lived alone and worked badly in a job she hated. Almost everyone was an enemy: her neighbours inflicted their noise and domestic quarrels on her; her employer criticised her shoddy timekeeping; her successful, cheerful colleagues had been corrupted by the system; attractive women had sold out to male chauvinism; only animals were faithful. She had one female friend with whom she had an alliance against the world. Together they would tease and torment any man who had the temerity to approach them. She was touchy and proud, terrified of humiliation, but also full of self-loathing, convinced that no one could ever love her.

She was 25 when she began psychotherapy three times a week; progress was very slow. At first any hint of hope was crushingly annihilated. She remained insistent that her life had been ruined by circumstances beyond her control, all was lost, there was no point in fighting for any improvement – better to make life intolerable for as many people as possible. If she must suffer, at least she could have the satisfaction of making other people, including her therapist, suffer as well.

In short, she made her life a monument to the grievance she held against people in authority in general, and against her father in particular. Never mind how much it hurt her, she would not give him the satisfaction of having a happy, successful daughter – that would be tantamount to forgiveness, which he absolutely did not deserve. Each year on the anniversary of her grandmother's death her depression intensified and, with the progress of mourning, the beloved grandmother came alive in the transference. Fitfully at first, her sessions could sometimes be a place where she could relax and feel accepted. She could begin to hope for change. This hopeful mood would be rapidly swept away by fresh waves of hatred and despair, when she felt her therapist failed her in one of the many ways that were possible. Holiday breaks were a torment since the therapist could not be trusted to return alive, nor could she be forgiven for giving her patient such a fright.

However, notwithstanding the awful danger of coming alive, she set about applying for the university course she had always wanted to do. With university came friendships, rivalry and betrayal, success and failure. Her alliance with her man-hating friend dissolved as she recognised the perversity and cruelty of their crusade. Tentatively she fell in love and was very painfully disappointed. But she forgave. She even contacted and visited her father, the first time in 15 years.

Six years of psychotherapy ended because she felt ready for independence. She believed psychotherapy had helped her reclaim her life, she was in no doubt that there would be further struggles, but she felt incomparably enriched by the experience.

Discussion

These four cases are drawn from my own NHS practice. In each case the intervention made a difference, allowing the people concerned to move on in their lives. Their capacities to work and to love more effectively, and with satisfaction, had been significantly enhanced. How is it that such very different interventions were required to obtain apparently rather similar results?

Sudden change is the most difficult to investigate or to explain. Miss B's change of heart was quite unexpected. In their letter at follow-up, her parents indicated that their daughter had continued to struggle with anxiety symptoms at times of increased stress, but had persevered successfully. However, they remained protective of her, apparently fearing she might relapse. What had proved so potent about a single family meeting?

The case of Mr and Mrs A. is rather easier to understand. The couple were in crisis, having taken on a major challenge. Both parties had vulnerabilities on account of their past experiences and were more angry and disappointed with each other than they were able to admit. In their case the therapist's main contribution was to find a way of saying, on behalf of each member of the couple, the things they had been trying ineffectually to say to one another, in a way that the other could at last hear.

This unblocked communication between them. They were both able and willing to forgive and try again.

Essentially, brief interventions must work by unblocking an impasse in communication, either between family members or within the mind of a single person, in such a way that already existing capacities for thoughtful co-operation become available once more to the persons involved. In each of the first two examples it is arguable that actions had taken over from words as a means of communication and that actions have the disadvantage of being more readily misinterpreted. From a psychoanalytic perspective, the key members of each family became locked in a repetitive pattern or enactment (Hinshelwood, 1987), in which each had their established role from which they were unable to escape, and which at an unconscious level provided sufficient gratification of certain unconscious impulses or fantasies, embedded in the enactment, so as to offset the disadvantages of the obviously painful malady that the repetitive drama represented. This formulation draws upon Freud's suggestion that a symptom or symptomatic action contains within it both the gratification of a forbidden wish and a punishment for it, in a symbolic form.

For example, in the second case one could speculate that for Miss B.'s family the conflict was over a reworking of the Oedipal situation: Miss B.'s preoccupation with her (to her own eyes) inadequate appearance may have been covering up the triumph she unconsciously felt over her mother, whom she may have assumed was envious of her youth and beauty, while she stole her father away on a wild-goose chase. By defeating him she may have been countering incestuous wishes that were too close for comfort, though her excited contempt for his efforts suggests a triumphant attack on her parents as an effective couple. Adolescents engaged in reworking Oedipal conflicts inevitably reawaken such conflicts for their parents, who are then faced with the challenge of reworking them too (Pincus and Dare, 1978). Possibly for Mrs B. it was unconsciously less painful to have a neurotic daughter, who could not enjoy her youthful beauty, than to accept the fact that her own reproductive life was nearing its end, though consciously she wanted her daughter to be a credit to her. In a way Mr B. could keep his daughter, thereby denying the passage of time and advancing age, though consciously the last thing he wanted was the continuing anxiety of a suicidal young woman.

Of course, this formulation has to remain speculative since none of the family has been subjected to psychoanalytic scrutiny. However, supposing it or something similar were the case, the enactment can only be sustained if a number of shared assumptions go unchallenged. In other words, it only works in the service of unconscious fantasy as a closed system of ideas. Since the intervention was effective, albeit unintentionally, we are entitled to assume that some shared assumptions were challenged. A new perspective on these assumptions may have opened somebody's eyes to the absurdity of the situation, someone may have felt ridiculous or ashamed, someone may have looked ahead. The balance of opinion between Mr and Mrs B. may have shifted such that Mr B. was better able to listen to his wife so that they could function more effectively as a couple.

According to this view, the repetitive patterns serve to protect each member of the family from unwelcome reality, either internal (fantasy) or external. The closed system of assumptions is closed against these realities, setting up an alternative set of propositions to which everyone agrees. Since these propositions are expressed through action, each individual's interpretation of them can remain unarticulated. Thus, it is possible for assumptions to be only apparently shared: each person may actually be holding an interpretation of events that contradicts that of others, but since none of the interpretations are expressed verbally, the assumptions are treated as if they are shared. As their function is the avoidance of psychic pain, these closed systems are difficult to challenge. We are all susceptible to signals, operating subliminally or unconsciously, warning us not to rock the boat. Participation in a defensive enactment greatly reduces the possibility of learning from experience. This accounts for the 'crisis of stuckness' that brought the first two cases in search of help. In view of their responsiveness to relatively minor interventions, upon which they were able to build, for each individual there must have been a balance in favour of respecting reality.

When are brief interventions not enough?

What of the person whose impasse has become a way of life? Both Miss J. and Miss K. were young women who had serious difficulties in sustaining loving and co-operative relationships and in applying themselves to work with any degree of satisfaction. For each of them, in different ways, the world was a hostile place which, only too predictably, fulfilled their expectations of hurt and disappointment. Both were willing to acknowledge that their trouble was now their own responsibility, whatever their view of its origins, and both unwillingly accepted that they needed professional help. For both of them the psycho-therapeutic encounter required courage and perseverance, at times they hated and feared it, but eventually both had the generosity to acknowledge the benefit of it. How was this achieved?

There are, of course, many differences in the detail of their progress, but something they had in common was the way that their descriptions of their daily experiences slowly changed: the number of helpful, friendly people they met slowly increased, they gradually began to believe they were not automatically disbarred from achieving what they wanted. Although still experiencing set-backs as major disasters, they developed some resilience in picking themselves up and trying again.

One might almost believe that the patient's luck had changed, and, as the therapy progressed, one had cause to be grateful to the new people in their lives who seemed to be reinforcing the therapeutic process. This was not a smooth development, there were inevitably set-backs and false hopes, yet an important criterion for being able to end the therapy was the sense that each woman had a number of trustworthy friends with whom future development was a possibility. In other words, they had reached a position through the therapeutic process that, it is postulated, was already available, though temporarily inaccessible, to the individuals in the first two examples.

Naturally, no one would in reality claim that psychotherapy changes a person's luck, so how does this change occur and why does it not happen spontaneously? This is a question that has occupied psychoanalysts since Freud first discovered the phenomenon of resistance. He began with the optimistic assumption that patients would be pleased to learn the truth about themselves, if it meant that they would be relieved of their symptoms. Instead it is often the case that truth is repudiated as patients turn to their symptoms as a drowning man to a life-raft. This led Freud to describe the negative therapeutic reaction (1923) and to his theory of the death instinct (1920). He regarded the compulsion to repeat, observable in the transference, as a manifestation of a fundamental conservatism in human nature, reflecting a preference for no pain, no disturbance, nothing new or challenging.

In *Two Principles of Mental Functioning* (1911) he called this conservative tendency the Pleasure Principle. It is opposed by the Reality Principle, without which life would not be sustainable. As Bion (1962*a,b*) observed, Truth or Reality is as necessary for mental development as food is for the body. Martha Harris (1968, p. 8) quotes a boy whose analysis involved a prolonged and violent period of resistance as saying 'Why should finding out that I am such a bastard make me feel so much better?' This was after a prolonged struggle on his part not to hear the truth about himself as he heaped scorn upon his analyst.

Our understanding of this phenomenon has evolved through the work of Melanie Klein (1975) and those who have further elaborated her theory (Spillius, 1988). She describes two main types of anxiety that must be faced during normal development; that associated with the Paranoid–Schizoid position, which has to do with the threat of annihilation of the self and that associated with the Depressive position which has to do with the survival of the person(s) upon whom one depends for succour and sustenance. She extended Freud's theory of the Death Instinct by proposing that the source of both types of anxiety lies in innate destructive impulses.

Klein observed that young children can employ a kind of mental resting place, which she called the manic defence, in which there is a radical denial of internal reality, and to some extent of external reality, on the basis of identification with an idealised omnipotent figure. Here the child is free of both paranoid and depressive anxiety since he feels invulnerable and in need of no one. Envy is abolished. Ordinarily this is a transient state that is terminated by the breaking through of such realities as hunger, pain, exhaustion, etc. However, in unduly adverse circumstances this manic defence becomes a safe haven, protected by an elaborate system of defences, which effect a more or less stable compromise (through misrepresentation) with reality. Anna Freud's (1936) defence 'Identification with the aggressor' would be an example of a stable derivative of the manic position through the elaboration of sado-masochistic fantasy which may or may not be the result of a traumatic experience.

Psychotherapy and relinquishing Psychic Retreats

Steiner (1993) has suggested that we all have recourse to such a 'Psychic Retreat' when faced with a sufficiently severe challenge to our psychic integrity, but that some patients, typically those who are difficult to treat, spend much of their time in this mental place. His extensive clinical observations have led him to propose that the construction of a psychic retreat, or defensive organisation (O'Shaughnessy, 1981), is based upon setting up a perverse relation to reality. He suggests that the psychic retreat masquerades as a good and protective place, but actually contains such an admixture of cruelty and tyranny that it keeps the dependent and potentially healthy part of the self in thrall. He observes that there is often a seductive or addictive relationship between the dependent self and the various fantasies that underpin the complex of defences of the psychic retreat.

Of course, the more this system of defences is employed, the more difficult it becomes to face the reality outside: the waste and destruction wreaked both internally and externally under cover of the defensive fantasies. The safe haven is ever more desperately endorsed: 'There is no alternative!' This, by the way, offers an explanation for personality deterioration over time.

Against such a powerful system, ordinary, mutually dependent human relationships have a hard time recommending themselves. Under the onslaught of subtle travesties of reality the therapist strives to make contact with those aspects of the patient that, at least potentially, are able to recognise and flourish in the world of common shared reality. It could be argued that this was possible with both Miss J. and Miss K., but that the long duration of their treatments was because of their use of psychic retreats that only slowly yielded to the gradual strengthening of their links with a more benign, reality-oriented internal object, at least partially built by their experience of a containing therapist who was not intimidated or driven to despair by their retreat. The construction over time of an internal therapeutic alliance helped both women to recognise helpful figures in the external world and to work co-operatively with them.

It is not uncommon that patients find others, like Miss K.'s 'friend' who willingly bolster the false propositions of the psychic retreats. 'All men are hateful; victims are entitled to exploit the fortunate; drugs enhance consciousness; life is pointless; death is desirable.' Therapy is only viable if part of the patient is not convinced by falsity for part of the time. During those moments of escape one endeavours to sense and address the anxieties that drive the patient into retreat, offering an alternative, namely containment, to the attractions of the psychic retreat.

Put at its simplest, the proposition here is that in order for a person to be able to make use of brief psychotherapy the balance of forces within the personality must be in favour of the reality principle. That is, the patient has an internal model of healthy dependency, meaning a relationship in which there is mutual recognition of differences and a willingness to work together in the light of common shared reality. While this internal model may be temporarily unavailable to the person(s) concerned, because they have been caught up in a closed system of false propositions (whether shared or apparently shared), the brief therapeutic intervention has the effect of releasing curiosity, imagination and forgiveness in the service of resolving the present crisis. Successful resolution of crisis strengthens the person's confidence in the co-operative potential of human relations. An effective challenge to the misconceptions embedded in the symptomatic drama should to a degree lessen their hold on the mind.

However, no progress can be made if the balance of forces in mind is in favour of the pleasure principle. This does not mean that the person does not suffer, but that his suffering is in the service of obscuring reality (Riesenberg-Malcolm, 1981). For example, Rosenfeld (1964) has suggested that substance addiction is an attempt to shore up manic defences in flight from unbearable inner reality. According to this suggestion, the mental defences to which the addict has recourse are inadequate and he is drawn to even more destructive attacks on his reality sense by using drugs or alcohol. For such a person, psychoanalytic psychotherapy can pose a real danger, if the anxiety mobilised by the therapy cannot be effectively contained, since he may be driven back to drugs or substance abuse as a short term but reliable 'cure' for mental pain. This is not to say that ex-addicts cannot make good use of psychotherapy, only that extra care is required. For example, psychoanalytic psychotherapy may only be a viable option if there is a sufficiently strong supportive framework for the patient such as a day-hospital programme and trained staff who can respond effectively to a crisis.

As a general rule, one would recommend that, in any case, the initial psychotherapeutic approach should involve the family if possible. This is in accordance with Haley's (1980) hierarchy of hopefulness. It may be that by engaging with the family first, an impasse in communication could be unblocked thereby mobilising the constructive potential of all family members, including the patient. At the very least, close family members are entitled to be warned of the dangers of psychoanalytic psychotherapy for an abstinent ex-addict.

However, in the cases of Miss J. and Miss K., there was no prospect of approaching their families. They were both single and they positively did not want to involve family members. They did not present in crisis, but had for many years been trying to find the help they needed. Their relative isolation was their way of surviving, yet their survival was a burden to them. It would be false to say that they had no notion of healthy dependence as has been defined here. Indeed, at some level they longed for it, but it was not available to them because their inner reality was dominated by hostility, cruelty and suspicion. They had little confidence in other's good intentions, retreating instead to a citadel of defensive misconceptions. Yet for psychotherapy to have been a viable undertaking, each of them must have had sufficient respect for reality that a therapeutic alliance could be forged. On the basis of this, and of its vicissitudes, change was possible. It is not difficult to imagine how much more difficult an enterprise psychotherapy would have been if either of them had used drugs as a way of both reinforcing their psychic retreats, and of punishing their therapist.

References

Appelbaum, S. (1977) *The Anatomy of Change*. New York: Plenum.

Bion, W. R. (1962*a*) A theory of thinking. *International Journal of Psychoanalysis*, **43**, 306–10.

Bion, W. R. (1962*b*) *Learning from Experience*. London: Heineman.

Crits-Christoph, P. (1992) The efficacy of brief dynamic psychotherapy: a meta-analysis. *American Journal of Psychiatry*, **49**, 151–8.

Dahl, H., Kachele, H. and Thoma, H. (eds.) (1988) *Psychoanalytic Process Research Strategies*. Berlin, Heidelberg: Springer–Verlag.

Davanloo, H. (1978) *Basic Principles and Techniques in Short-Term Dynamic Psychotherapy: A Treatment Manual*. New York: Basic Books.

Freud, S. (1911) Two principles of mental functioning. In: Strachey, J. (ed.) *The Standard Edition of the Complete Psychological Works of Sigmund Freud*, Vol. 12, pp. 213–26. London: Hogarth Press.

Freud, A. (1936) *The Ego and Its Mechanisms of Defence*. London: Hogarth Press.

Freud, S. (1920) Beyond the pleasure principle. In: Strachey, J. (ed.) *The Standard Edition of the Complete Psychological Works of Sigmund Freud*, Vol. 18, pp. 1–64. London: Hogarth Press.

Freud, S. (1923) The ego and the id. In: Strachey, J. (ed.) *The Standard Edition of the Complete Psychological Works of Sigmund Freud*, Vol. 19, pp. 1–66. London: Hogarth Press.

Frosch, S. (1987) *The Politics of Psycho-Analysis*. London: Macmillan.

Harris, M. (1958) The therapeutic process in the psychoanalytic treatment of the child. In: Harris Williams, M. (ed.) *Collected Papers of Martha Harris and Esther Bick*, pp. 3–17. Perthshire: Clunie Press (1987).

Haley, J. (1980 *Leaving Home*. New York: McGraw Hill.

Hinshelwood, R. D. (1987) *What Happens in Groups? Psychoanalysis, the Individual and the Community*. London: Free Associations Books.

Horowitz, L., (1974) *Clinical Prediction in Psychotherapy*. New York: Aronson.

Kernberg, O., Burstein, E., Coyne, L., Appelbaum, A., Horowitz, L. and Volter, H. (1972) Psychotherapy and psychoanalysis: final report of the Menniger Foundation's psychotherapy research project. *Bulletin of the Menniger Clinic*, **36**, 1–275.

Kernberg, O. F., Selzer, M. A., Koenigsburg, H. W., Caw, A. C. and Appelbaum, A. H (1989) *Psychodynamic Psychotherapy of Borderline Patients*. New York: Basic Books.

Klein, M. (1932) *The Psycho-Analysis of Children, The Writings of Melanie Klein*, Vol. 2. London: Hogarth Press (1975).

Klein, M. (1975) *The Writings of Melanie Klein*, Vols. 1–3 London: Hogarth Press.

Luborsky, L. (1984) *Principles of Psychoanalytic Psychotherapy: A Manual for Supportive Expressive Treatment*. New York: Basic Books.

Luborsky, L. and Crits-Christoph, P. (1990) *Understanding the Transference*. New York: Basic Books.

Luborsky, L., Crits-Christoph, P., Mints, J. and Auerbach, A. (1988) *Who Will Benefit from Psychotherapy? Predicting Therapeutic Outcomes*. New York: Basic Books.

Malan, D. H. (1963) *A Study of Brief Psychotherapy*. London: Tavistock Publications.

Malan, D. H. and Osimo, F. (1992) *Psychodynamics, Training and Outcome in Brief Psychotherapy*. London: Butterworth-Heineman Ltd.

Meissner, W. W. (1981) Addiction and paranoid process: Psychoanalytic perspectives. *International Journal of Psychoanalytic Psychotherapy*, **8**, 273–310.

Murray-Parkes, C., Stevenson-Hinde, J. and Marris, P. (eds.) (1991) *Attachment Across the Life-Cycle*. London: Routledge & Kegan Paul.

O'Shaughnessy, E. (1981) A clinical study of defensive organisation, *International Journal of Psycho-Analysis*, **62**, 359–69.

Pincus, L. and Dare, C. (1978) *Secrets in the Family*. London: Faber.

Riesenberg-Malcolm, R. (1981) Expiation as a defence. *International Journal of Psychoanalytic Psychotherapy*, **8**, 549–70.

Rosenfeld, H. A. (1960) On drug addiction. *International Journal of Psycho-Analysis*, **41**, 467–75.

Rosenfeld, H. A. (1964) *The Psychopathology of Drug Addiction and Alcoholism: A Critical Review of the Psycho-Analytic Literature in Psychotic States*. New York: International University Press.

Rosenfeld, H. A. (1965) *Psychotic States: A Psychoanalytic Approach*. London: Hogarth Press.

Rosenfeld, H. A. (1987) *Impasse and Interpretation*. London: Tavistock Publications.

Ryle, A. (1975) *Frames and Cages. The Repertory Grid Approach to Human Understanding*. Sussex University Press.

Ryle, A. (1990) *Cognitive-Analytic Therapy, Active Participation in Change*. London: Wiley.

Scharff, J. S. (ed.) (1985) *Foundations of Object Relations Family Therapy*. Northvale, N.J, London: Aronson.

Searles, H. F. (1965) *Collected Papers on Schizophrenia and Related Subjects*. London: Hogarth Press.

Sifneos, P. E. (1992) *Short-Term Anxiety Provoking Psychotherapy: A Treatment Manual*. New York: Basic Books.

Slipp, S. (1988) *The Technique and Practice of Object Relations Family Therapy*. Northvale, NJ, London: Aronson.

Smaldino, A. (ed.) (1991) *Psychoanalytic Approaches to Addiction*. New York: Brunner Mazel.

Spillius, E. B. (1983) Some Developments from the Work of Melanie Klein. *International Journal of Psycho-Analysis*, **41**, 467–75.

Spillius, E. B. (ed.) (1988) *Melanie Klein Today*. London: Routledge & Kegan Paul.

Steiner, J. (1993) *Psychic Retreats: Pathological Organisations in Psychotic, Neurotic and Borderline Patients*. London: Routledge & Kegan Paul.

Stern, D. N. (1985) *The Interpersonal World of the Human Infant.* New York: Basic Books.

Strupp, H. H. and Binder, J. L. (1984) *Psychotherapy in a New Key: A Guide to Time-Limited Dynamic Psychotherapy.* New York: Basic Books.

Wallerstein, R. (1986) *Forty-two Lives in Treatment: A Study of Psycho-analysis and Psychotherapy.* New York: Guilford.

Yorke, C. (1970) A critical review of some psychoanalytic literature on drug addiction. *British Journal of Medical Psycology*, **43**, 141–59.

6

Addictive behaviour: the next clinic appointment

GRIFFITH EDWARDS

Introduction

Dependence on alcohol or on other drugs, once established, constitutes a potentially malign condition. Consider, for example, results from a 20-year follow-up of 100 men with alcohol dependence (Marshall *et al.*, 1994), who at the study intake point had a mean age of 42. Twenty years later, 44% had died, with an observed/expected mortality ratio of 3.64. Seventeen per cent were still drinking in a dependent fashion and 17% were abstinent. The 11% who had achieved social drinking included subjects whose loss of tolerance or state of physical health now precluded anything but a moderate intake. If we were to apportion the 11% untraced equally between troubled and untroubled drinking, the data would suggest that 20 years subsequent to the study intake point almost exactly two-thirds of patients will be dead or still drinking in a destructive fashion, while one-third will be abstinent or have ameliorated their drinking. These results are much in line with previous findings, (for instance, those of Nicholls *et al.*, 1974; Edwards *et al.*, 1983; Vaillant, 1983; Berglund, 1984; Frances *et al.*, 1987).

If these data on alcohol dependence are worrying, they contrast favourably with parallel data from a 22-year follow-up that the National Addiction Centre has conducted on a cohort of 128 heroin users (Oppenheimer *et al.*, 1994). Subjects had a mean age of 26 years at study intake and at the follow-up the observed/expected mortality ratio was something over 12. In other words, these young addicts faced twelve times the mortality expectation of their non-addict contemporaries. This study overlapped with, but largely predated, the HIV era, and HIV is in the long-term likely to add significantly to the mortality experience of injecting drug users. Other studies from a number of

94

different countries confirm the seriousness of opiate dependence (Vaillant, 1973; Murphy, 1988; Rossow, 1994; Marx *et al.*, 1994).

Thus, by any reckoning, substance dependence is a worrying, life-threatening condition. We and our patients are playing for high stakes and it must surely behove us to meet our responsibilities by getting the best possible treatment in place for each patient, and as early as possible.

But what is for any given patient 'the best possible treatment'? We are, of course, concerned here with a wide range of patients and problems. There is also a broad choice of treatments from which to make a selection, delivered in the in-patient or out-patient setting, and with greater or lesser intensity of treatment input (Kleber, 1989; Saunders, 1989; Institute of Medicine, 1990). Furthermore, different patients may respond selectively to different types of intervention, although support for the so-called 'matching hypothesis' (Glaser, 1980) is not conclusive (Edwards and Taylor, 1994). We will not deal here with primary health care strategies directed at early problem drinking (Babor *et al.*, 1986; Bien *et al.*, 1993).

At our various clinics or community centres, or on our hospital wards, whatever our country, will be some patients who are doing rewardingly well, others for whom it is still too early to detect much progress, and still others who are finding the going difficult. To make the abstract quest for 'best possible treatment' real, let's humanise the question and look at the problem as set by a patient of a kind who might be found at any alcohol problems clinic, any day, in many different countries.

At the time of referral, about five years ago, Mrs Able (a cover name for a real person) was aged 35, a highly proficient branch manager of a large supermarket chain. Abnormal liver function tests were picked up at a routine health screening and hence a referral to the clinic. Mrs Able was always markedly well dressed, confident, charming, and tense. Her husband was a successful executive. They had at the time of referral a teenage son and a daughter, who were both winning prizes at school, and their home was in a pleasant, leafy suburb. The history of this confident woman was of a childhood home marked by an ineffectual father and a heavily drinking, chaotic mother. The mother, now severely brain damaged, was still alive, and Mrs Able would go round and see her each week, consumed on each occasion by feelings of pity, and a rage of hatred. Mrs Able herself, however, after a hard and sober day's work had now for several years been in the habit of getting home at 7 p.m., and by 9 p.m. she would usually be blind drunk, falling over, and passing out in her elegant suburban home, to the distress, confusion, anger, and disgust of her family.

Let's see how a debate around Mrs Able's story can be used to test and clarify our latent beliefs as to the nature of the disorder from which our patients are suffering, with the consequent follow-through from specification of disorder, to the chosen model of treatment.

What we will now venture upon is an exploration of ideas. The intention is to explore the broad, underlying, beliefs which shape our therapeutic responses to patients who are dependent on alcohol or drugs. The exploration of ideas is always a dangerous business, easily becoming too speculative or grandiose. However, one might argue that in any research group or clinical centre, it is vital to find time to ask what we are *really* doing, what we *really* believe, what are the covert assumptions that shape our treatments, and where do we stand in the face of history (Levine, 1978; Berridge, 1993).

So what do we really think is wrong with Mrs Able? In simplified terms, an analysis of the nature of Mrs Able's problem might be seen as likely to take us in one of two broad directions. Firstly, there is the view that this patient's fundamental problem is at the psychodynamic level and resides in her being, with her drinking only the outward manifestation of her disturbance in relationship with self and others, or in shorthand terms the problem is her neurosis. Secondly, there is the approach that sees the priority issue as the drug-seeking or alcohol-seeking behaviour. From those contrasting conceptual formulations will logically flow vastly different ideas as to the appropriate models for individual treatment, the organisation of treatment services, and the nature of the requisite professional training.

We have here a conflict in belief that won't go away even if we choose to ignore it. Many treatment and research centres fail to clarify where they position themselves in this debate, and hope just to muddle along. The clinicians may continue to treat their patients in therapeutic groups where the essential assumptions are dynamic, while the treatment research concentrates on biological and behavioural approaches that are blind to dynamics. An anthropologist visiting our centres would find it difficult to identify, as it were, what gods we worship. We would probably all argue that at the end of the day a degree of eclecticism is often likely to be the best answer. However, eclecticism will be only a muddle rather than a useful compromise, if differing positions are not first defined and tested. At worst, a thoughtless compromise may be no more than a fusion of errors.

Substance dependence as neurosis: the theoretical postulate

Let's now look in a little more detail at the first of these two broad alternative views, and visit if not worship at the temple of Freud. A brief survey of statements made on substance misuse by psychoanalysts and other practitioners of dynamic psychotherapy reveals several variations around a core explanation of the problem in terms of neurosis and childhood trauma. Here are some quotations by way of example:

Effective treatment of alcoholism must address the core problem of the alcoholic, namely, the enormous difficulties that such people have had in controlling and regulating their behaviour, feelings, and self-esteem.

(Khantzian, 1981)

Oral fixation is thought to be the arrested stage of development in the alcoholic. This fixation accounts for infantile and dependent characteristics such as narcissism, demanding behaviour, passivity, and dependence.

(Zimberg, 1985)

Orally addictive persons (alcoholics, compulsive overeaters, prescription and other 'pill' addicts, and heavy marijuana smokers), have experienced intense anxiety within the context of their mothering relationships during their initial weeks and months of life . . . In essence, the addict is a person who has experienced intense and chronic early-life anxiety as a result of prototaxically fearing destruction and annihilation by significant others.

(Forrest, 1985)

The feature linking those statements is the assumption that these patients constitute a distinct category of persons, characterised by a deficit that is fundamental and pervasive and of psychodynamic nature, and rooted in early relationships. What do we today make of these analytical formulations? Some of us might confess to finding the language in which they are written a little jarring. These statements seem perhaps too confident, too all-embracing, a dressing up of mystery in fine words. There is a tendency towards stereotyping and a vision of our patient as people not like us, and yet we should acknowledge that these quotations derive from experienced practitioners who have worked with many patients over many years. Confronted by Mrs Able, we might feel that we have something to learn from them, even if we do not share their pure faith or light candles at their shrines. But is this dynamic formulation in any sense a conjecture capable of refutation?

An assertion of this kind is probably only to a limited extent testable by scientific method. One can, however, approach the matter by examining whether there is any objective evidence that therapy based on the presumed validity of these psychodynamic formulations can give positive results. That would be a way of testing the underlying assumptions, at least obliquely. There are three types of data that we might wish to consider as potentially bearing on that question.

Firstly, we might try to determine the efficacy of psychotherapy for substance misuse through review of controlled trials on treatment of drinking problems. Here one discovers that insight-oriented psychotherapy for alcohol dependence has been rated as ineffective on the evidence of an influenced analysis of the alcohol treatment literature conducted by Miller and Hester (1986). However, if one goes back and looks at the primary material that was available to these authors as basis for their review, it is possible to derive a conclusion other than the one that they themselves draw. It is not really so much a matter of such psychotherapy having been proved to be worthless (an over-interpretation of the literature), but more a matter of the specific question never having so far been put satisfactorily to the test of controlled trial. Research that provides a clean test and with adequate power for the efficacy of any modern version of short-term (say six months) psychotherapy applied to alcohol problems has seemingly not been reported, and there is thus still a crucial gap in the literature. Given the strong general tradition that has now been established in psychotherapy research, this situation seems surprising.

Turning to evidence from trials on the treatment of opiate misuse, interesting contributions have been made in this area over recent years by investigators working in New Haven and Philadelphia who have reported a series of studies focusing on the added advantage that may be gained if some kind of counselling or psychotherapy is combined wth methadone in the treatment of opiate dependence (Woody *et al.*, 1983, 1987; Luborsky *et al.*, 1985; Carroll and Rounsaville, 1993). When interpreting this research one is, though, immediately confronted by the question of what is to be meant by 'psychotherapy'. Interpersonal psychotherapy, supportive expressive therapy, cognitive behavioural therapy, and counselling, were the treatment modalities that were assessed by these investigators within the frame of several linked controlled trials using similar methodologies. There were no control groups that received methadone alone. The main findings of this work can be summarised thus. First, whether any specific psychotherapy did better than counselling was likely to depend on the quality of the counselling, and if the counselling was well conducted it could achieve results equal to those obtained with one of the more sophisticated approaches. Second, psychotherapy improved the ability of patients with high global ratings of psychiatric disturbance, high depression, or combination of depression with personality disturbance, to benefit from methadone. Third, there were significant differences in effectiveness between therapists. A significant predictor of successful outcome was the patient's rating of the helping relationship, and this provided a stronger pointer than therapist compliance with treatment protocols.

Further research that may cast some light on the efficacy of treatment, which is modelled on the belief that it is the underlying neurosis that should be the treatment target, comes from a long-term follow-up of male alcoholics. Vaillant, in his *The Natural History of Alcoholism* (Vaillant, 1983), reported on two different follow-up populations. One sample recruited 400 youths from a poor inner city area and from a background that made subsequent access to psychotherapy limited. The second sample recruited 186 men on the basis of their enrolment at a prestigious East Coast American university, and these latter subjects would enter a culture and an income bracket in which over the 40-year follow-up period dynamic psychotherapy was readily available. One gets the feeling that in certain parts of America over that period, seeing an analyst was as ordinary as visiting a dentist. This second follow-up group therefore provided an important 'experiment of nature', for in many other cultures and epochs psychotherapy has been a commodity in distinctly more limited supply. With this group, which for the most part could be expected to pay for psychotherapy and which moved in a world where analysts were in abundance, and for those among these subjects who developed drinking problems, what was to be the observed relationship between engagement in psychotherapy and recovery from drinking?

Let's look at Vaillant's findings, which are, of course, epidemiological rather than of an experimental or controlled nature. Among the 400 subjects from the inner city sample, 110 at some time experienced problems with drinking, and 8% at some time received psychotherapy. Among the 26 subjects in the College sample who developed alcohol problems, 17 (62%) received psychotherapy – psychotherapy was a class-related experience. Vaillant further reported that 'Among the 26 alcohol abusers in the College sample, at least 10 men received 100 hours of individual psychotherapy and collectively the 26 men received over 5000 hours'.

As regards the observed association between psychotherapy and drinking outcome, Vaillant reported as follows:

. . . for only 2 College men was such therapy significantly associated with abstinence or return to asymptomatic drinking. One of these 2 men relapsed and is
now a member of AA.

The sample of College problem drinkers that Vaillant studied was
relatively small. Nonetheless there is evidence here of significant relevance to our quest for information that can help us decide whether we
should be referring Mrs Able to analytical psychotherapy. There is nothing in Vaillant's findings to make us feel that we will be failing in our
responsibilities to our patients if we do not route Mrs Able to intensive
dynamic psychotherapy, or to suggest that a person with a drinking
problem who lives in a city with many analysts is more fortunate than
someone living in an environment where analysts are not too thick on the
ground.

So where does the evidence seem to lead in relation to questions about
a model of treatment based on the assumption that the problem is not the
peripheral symptom, but rather the core neurotic disorder resident within
that person? The question will not go away, but it is not at present one
that in objective scientific terms is capable of strict answer. The scientific
fashions of the day might lead us to assume that dynamically based
therapy for substance problems should properly be viewed as dead or
discredited, but that is in reality as much an unscientific position as the
claim that dynamic psychotherapy, group or individual, is known to
work. What one might take away from this inevitably brief attempt to
examine a difficult question is a set of three conclusions. Firstly, one
might wish to form an alliance with a research-minded psychotherapist
who is expert in brief, focused dynamic psychotherapy of a modern kind,
and carry out a control trial – such research would be timely and greatly
welcomed by the treatment community. Secondly, there is the hint from
O'Brien and Woody's research that the therapeutic relationship is a predictor of outcome, a hint of a dynamic kind. Thirdly, from Vaillant's
clever exploitation of an experiment of nature there is the message that
intensive, prolonged, conventional psychotherapy of an analytical variety
is unlikely to be good medicine for substance problems. Vaillant has
argued this same view elsewhere (Vaillant, 1981). Finally, under this
heading we had better again admit that we are searching around for
hints and murmurs while the obvious and needed research remains unap-
proached. But an encounter with Mrs Able, watching her face as she talks
about her mother, is likely to reawaken interest in these questions. Some
people seem very much posessed by their past, with their drinking part of
a complex, shadowy, painful, self-entrapping play.

The behaviour as the problem

As already suggested, the major alternative to the postulate that the problem lies in an underlying psychodynamic disorder is the assumption that the priority problem is the substance-seeking behaviour itself (Miller and Heather, 1986). Within this latter formulation, Mrs Able's problem is not her conflicted identification with her mother or her acting out on her husband of childhood experience with her father, but the cues, cognitions and expectancies that will again provoke her drinking when she walks into her home this evening. The therapeutic approaches that flow from this latter conception are, then, likely to be based on multiple strategies that target multiple aspects of the present behaviour or particular circumscribed cognitions. Let's look in brief and selectively at just three types of approach that may contribute to the repertoire of interventions that derive from this behavioural definition of the problem.

Drug substitution

Methadone maintenance is a treatment approach that derives rationally from the postulate that heroin taking is a behaviour driven by the learning mechanisms that are inherent in opiate dependence. If the synthetic, oral, and more long-acting methadone is substituted for heroin, the need for an opiate will be met, drug-seeking behaviour curtailed, and the dangerous and socially disruptive injecting habit obviated. A behaviour is here being treated by pharmacotherapeutic means, and it is certainly the behaviour rather than any postulated neurosis that is the target. The results are likely to be influenced by sample selection and the quality of the treatment programme, but there is rather persuasive research evidence to support the effectiveness of methadone in curtailing needle use, enhancing social stability, and decreasing acquisitive crime (Ball and Ross, 1991). There is also evidence from a number of controlled trials to support the efficacy of nicotine substitution as treatment for cigarette smoking, using gum or patch (Foulds, 1993; Stapleton *et al.*, 1995). Effective pharmacotherapies are beginning to evolve for alcohol dependence (O'Malley *et al.*, 1992). For our present analysis what needs to be noted is not only the empirical fact that such treatments may confer advantage, but the underlying conceptual and theoretical implications that stem from these findings. At least in some circumstances the destructive consequences of substance-seeking behaviour may be ameliorated not by an approach that goes for deep interpersonal or intrapersonal causes, but by an approach that targets behaviour with a chemical bullet. We have left behind the blind blanketing of dependent patients with sedatives and tranquillisers, and today our chemotherapies are scientifically rational, and our missiles, as it were, increasingly smart.

The psychological extinction of relapse-provoking cues

The theoretical analysis underlying this treatment approach postulates that one reason why treated patients relapse is that they re-enter a world in which there are many cues that through learning processes will either precipitate a direct desire for drink or drugs, or provoke a conditioned withdrawal-like experience (Rosenow *et al.*, 1991). Extinction of such learning through a cue exposure and response prevention paradigm would on that analysis appear to be a rational treatment (Marlatt, 1990; Monti *et al.*, 1993). In practical terms this might, for instance, mean repeated sessions conducted in a safe therapeutic environment in which a patient would be invited to handle and sniff alcohol without drinking it. As with psychotherapy, so too in this instance there are possibilities for testing the validity of an underlying theory by examining the efficacy of a theory-derived treatment. If cue exposure treatment is a crucial test for the adequacy of a behavioural view of the addiction, the answers that it gives back are at present interesting but not conclusive. There is, however, a space here to be watched.

The community reinforcement approach

Here we turn from pharmacotherapy or behavioural treatment to an examination of what can be achieved by manipulation of the environment. Hunt and Azrin conducted a controlled evaluation of an approach in which patients with drinking problems were offered access to various privileges, including assistance with job finding and leisure rewards, contingent on sobriety. Four different trials of this general strategy have given positive results with the conceptual implication that dependent behaviour can be influenced by the reinforcing consequences that stem from change in behaviour (Azrin *et al.*, 1982; Sisson and Azrin, 1989).

We have discussed above just three selected examples of lines of research that support strategy of potential benefit. There is, of course, a far wider literature from which further evidence bearing on this debate could be drawn, including research on other types of pharmacological treatment (disulfiram and naltrexone, for instance) and other types of cognitive or behavioural treatment. Teaching of coping skills, aversion treatment, and motivational interviewing are examples (Marlatt and Gordon, 1985; Miller and Rollnick, 1991; Rollnick *et al.*, 1993), together with certain types of problem-oriented family therapy (Bennum, 1991). Approaches that focus on the behaviour might to those with an interest in psychodynamics appear banal, and even inhumane but, at least in terms of relatively short-term outcome, there is a confluence of research to suggest that a treatment approach that takes the behaviour as the salient problem has some underpinning. We would be foolish to take a hard, absolutist, partisan line, but that is today the general direction in which the evidence points.

Back to Mrs Able

Let's now return to the problem set by Mrs Able. It could be argued that her drinking is intensively cued to time of day, a certain setting, tiredness, a day's work accomplished, a sense of let-down. Anyone interested in family systems would offer yet another perspective. Her presentation also appears to be loaded with psychodynamic colouring. What will her fate be in 20 years time? After three years of eclectic treatment that used counselling, a low-key cognitive behavioural approach, attempts to persuade Mrs Able to affiliate to AA and with her husband also given some help, this patient showed no improvement whatsoever. Her psychiatrist seemed to have been rendered as ineffectual as the father who could not control the mother's drinking, or the husband whom Mrs Able reduced to tears. It was tempting to argue that the surface approach to the problem seen as the behaviour had failed, while we had neglected the deeper problems of the traumatised childhood, the existential pain, the purposive nature of the destruction of self and others, the 'neurosis', to use that old-fashioned word. With those data in mind, which tell us that at best Mrs Able has only a 33% chance of a good outcome, there is an anxious sense of time running out. At this sort of difficult frontline how is the research literature really to help with practical decision-making?

Let's at this juncture bring in just one further line of research evidence. The data in this instance derive from the same cohort of alcohol-dependent patients as provided those 20-year follow-up data quoted earlier (Edwards *et al.*, 1987). The results that we will now examine report the answers given to a structured questionnaire on patient attributions of cause for positive change in drinking behaviour, which was administered at ten-year follow-up to 66 of the surviving 80 patients, and these findings will again and in another context be considered in Chapter 14. We were thus asking patients themselves what they saw as the factors that brought about any degree of beneficial change within a ten-year time perspective, an approach that has both its strengths and its limitations. This material was later submitted to a principle-components analysis. Here let's report some raw scores. We are looking at an attribution rather than proven causality. Out of 70 items rated on a 5-point scale by these 66 patients, the following five items achieved the highest positive endorsement scores:

1. Wanting my self-respect (54% positive).
2. Determination not be be beaten by drink (54%).
3. What a psychiatrist said or did (53%).
4. Deciding my fate was in my own hands (53%).
5. Understanding myself better (49%).

This group of items suggests that self-esteem, self-efficacy and self-understanding were perceived as related to recovery, with a psychiatrist's intervention also viewed as helpful. Other than for the element of psychiatric help, these lead elements in the ranking are not specifically about drinking avoidance strategies, enhancement of coping skills, relapse prevention strategies, cue exposure, the readjustment of external influences, or interpersonal relationships, but are centrally about personal and inner change.

If we let our patients speak, they have something to tell. Change in the way patients feel about themselves, self-empowerment, a belief in the possibility of change, some optimism, may be vital ingredients of recovery in the long run. Again, this is a matter to which we will return in Chapter 14 when considering what may be learnt from Alcoholics Anonymous.

Toward a therapeutic synthesis

Back to Mrs Able. We have got to get on with her treatment, setting out the programme in the light of the research that is available, with open admission of the current research gaps. We might conjecture, and we can do no more than as best possible conjecture, that the best therapeutic formula within which to operate might be defined within a framework that tries to synthesise certain insights from the dynamic tradition with the problem-oriented approach, rather than putting the two conceptions in sharp opposition. Here is a provisional sketch of what such a framework might look like.

1. Our current and dominant therapeutic approach in this field is likely to concentrate as a priority on bringing about and supporting behavioural change in alcohol- or drug-taking. Understanding of motivation, cognitions and learning process is relevant to this intention. This approach offers a therapeutic perspective radically different to the orthodox analytical search for deep causes, but carries a risk of losing sight of the whole person.

2. The therapist at best supports natural processes of recovery, the natural helping processes (see p. 61). That may at times mean the sensitive, cautious, covert, nudging, deployment of psychodynamic insights.

3. Where dynamic understanding may further contribute to our work is by sensitising us to the realities and live possibilities of personal change toward autonomy, freedom, individualisation, self-understanding and altruism, so that we recognise, nurture, and reinforce these processes when we see them. The psychodynamic tradition rightly reminds us that life is about growth, and that recovery is a long play. We need to be aware of processes.

4. Finally, a general conclusion that brings together much that has been said above is the need for daily awareness that we are indeed ourselves active participants in the therapeutic play, and inescapably exposed to that responsibility. This may be one of the most important contributions the dynamic perspective can make. The first meeting with a patient has the capacity to enhance belief in the possibility of self-change (Thom *et al.*, 1992); ten years later, 'what a psychiatrist said or did' may be ranked highly as having contributed to change (Edwards *et al.*, 1987), and the American drugs research indicates that the therapist's qualities may be more important than the niceties of the treatment manual (Carrol and Rounsaville, 1993). We need to change and enhance our own effectiveness as change-agents.

So what happened next to Mrs Able? The usual approaches had, after three years, achieved little. She had broken contact and come back to see us again, and she and we felt that we were getting nowhere. At this point Mrs Able was referred for a specialist opinion to a very senior Kleinian analyst. She was, after assessment, accepted for psychotherapy. She decided to turn the offer down. If we felt that referral to psychotherapy was justified if only as a desperate throw of the dice, it was not a game of dice that she consented to play. Instead of entering psychotherapy, for the next year or so she continued to drink in a gradually worsening fashion. She was beginning to experience withdrawal symptoms. Her children no longer wanted to talk to her. There was trouble at work. After a particularly traumatic and drunken weekend her husband left home, moved into lodgings, and announced that he would start divorce proceedings. Mrs Able then stopped drinking, her husband returned to her, and 12 months later, at the time of writing, she is still sober. Perhaps some kind of turning point has been reached, and with continued sobriety will come other positive life changes, or perhaps that is all too optimistic and she will drink again next week. Perhaps the reason for her having for the first time attained any considerable period of sobriety is in part a sleeper effect of all our therapeutic inputs, or perhaps our efforts have nothing to do with this development. Perhaps she was responding purely and simply to the threat made by her husband, or perhaps that threat interacted with some deeper personal process of change. We can only go on working as best possible toward liberation of change.

Meanwhile, Mrs Able persuades us that in the difficult field in which we all labour, the path to a better future lies in a strong and continued relationship between the clinical and research worlds, the admission of doubt, and a commitment to listening to what our patients have to tell.

Acknowledgement

I am very grateful to Mrs Patricia Davies for her secretarial assistance.

References

Azrin, N. H., Sisson, R. W., Meyers, R. and Godley, M. (1982) Alcoholism treatment by disulfiram and community reinforcement therapy. *Journal of Behaviour Therapy and Experimental Psychiatry*, **13**, 105–12.

Babor, T. F., Ritson, E. B. and Hodgson, R. J. (1986) Alcohol-related problems in the primary health care setting: a review of early intervention strategies. *British Journal of Addiction*, **81**, 23–46.

Ball, J. C. and Ross, A. (1991) *The Effectiveness of Methadone Maintenance Treatment*. New York: Springer Verlag.

Bennun, I. (1991) Family therapy for alcohol problems. pp. 250–263. In: Glass, I. B. (ed.) *The International Handbook of Addiction Behaviour*, pp. 250–63. London: Routledge.

Berglund, M. (1984) Mortality in alcoholics related to clinical state at first admission. A study of 537 deaths. *Acta Psychiatrica Scandinavica*, **70**, 407–16.

Berridge, V. (1993) The nature of the target disorder: an historical perspective. In: Edwards, G., Strang, J. and Jaffe, J. H. (eds.) *Drugs, Alcohol and Tobacco: Making the Science and Policy Connections*, pp. 179–86. Oxford: OUP.

Bien, T., Miller, W. R. and Tannigan, S. (1993) Brief interventions for alcohol problems: A review. *Addiction*, **88**, 315–36.

Carroll, K. M. and Rounsaville, B. J. (1993) Implications of recent research on psychotherapy for drug abuse. In: Edwards, G., Strang, J. and Jaffe, J. H. (eds.) *Drugs, Alcohol and Tobacco: Making the Science and Policy Connections*, pp. 210–21. Oxford: OUP.

Edwards, G., Brown, D., Dukitt, A., Oppenheimer, E., Sheehan, M. and Taylor, C. (1987) Outcome of alcoholism: the structure of patient attributions as to what causes change. *British Journal of Addiction*, **82**, 533–45.

Edwards, G., Oppenheimner, E., Duckitt, A., Sheehan, M. and Taylor, C. (1983) What happens to alcoholics? *Lancet* **ii**, 269–71.

Edwards, G. and Taylor C. (1994) A test of the matching hypothesis: alcohol dependence, intensity of treatment, and 12 month outcome. *Addiction*, **89**, 553–61.

Forrest, G. G. (1985) Psychodynamically oriented treatment of alcoholism and substance abuse. In: Bratter, T. E. and Forrest, G. G. (eds.) *Alcoholism and Substance Abuse: Strategies for Clinical Intervention*, pp. 307–36. New York: Free Press.

Foulds, J. (1993) Does nicotine replacement therapy work? *Addiction*, **88**, 1473–8.

Frances, R. J., Franklin, J. and Flarin, D. K. (1987) Suicide and alcoholism. *American Journal of Drug and Alcohol Abuse*, **13**, 327–41.

Glaser, F. B. (1980) Anybody got a match? Treatment research and the matching hypothesis. In: Edwards, G. and Grant, M. (eds.) *Alcoholism Treatment in Transition*, pp. 178–96. London: Croon Helm.

Institute of Medicine (1990) *Broadening the Base of Treatment for Alcohol Problems*. Washington DC: National Academy Press.

Khantzian, W. J. (1981) Some treatment implications of the ego and self-disturbance in alcoholism. In: Bean, M. H. and Zimberg, N. E. (eds.) *Dynamic Approaches to the Understanding and Treatment of Alcoholism*, pp. 163–88. Free Press: New York.

Kleber, H. D. (1989) Treatment of drug dependence: What works. *International Review of Psychiatry*, **1**, 81–100.

Levine, H. G. (1978) The discovery of alcoholism: changing perceptions of habitual drunkenness in American history. *Journal of Studies on Alcohol*, **39**, 143–74.

Luborsky, L., McLellan, A. J., Woody, G. E., O'Brien, C. P. and Anerback, A. (1985) Therapist success and its determinants. *Archives of General Psychiatry*, **42**, 602–11.

Marlatt, G. A. (1990) Cue exposure and relapse prevention in the treatment of addictive behaviors. *Addictive Behaviors*, **15**, 359–9.

Marlatt, G. A. and Gordon, J. A. (1985) *Relapse Prevention*. New York: Guilford Press.

Marshall, E. J., Edwards, G. and Taylor, C. (1994) Mortality in men with drinking problems: a 20 year follow-up. *Addiction*, **89**, 1293–8.

Marx, A., Schlick, M. T. and Minder, C. E. (1994) Drug-related mortality in Switzerland from 1987–1989 in comparison to other countries. *International Journal of the Addictions*, **29**, 837–60.

Miller, W. R. and Heather, N. (eds.) (1986) *Treating Addictive Behaviours: Processes of Change*. New York: Plenum.

Miller, W. R. and Hester, R. K. (1986) The effectiveness of alcoholism treatment: what research reveals. In: Miller, W. R. and Heather, N. (eds.) *Treating Addictive Behaviours: Processes of Change*, pp. 121–74. New York: Plenum.

Miller, W. R. and Rollnick, S. (1991) Motivational interviewing: preparing people to change. In: *Addictive Behaviour*. New York: Guilford.

Monti, P. M., Rohsenow, D. J. Rubonis, A. V. *et al.* (1993) Cue exposure with coping skills training for male alcoholics: a preliminary investigation. *Journal of Consulting and Clinical Psychology*, **61**, 1011–19.

Murphy, G. E. (1988) Suicide and substance abuse. *Archives of General Psychiatry*, **65**, 593–4.

Nicholls, P., Edwards, G. and Kyle, E. (1974) Alcoholics admitted to four hospitals in England II. General and cause-specific mortality. *Quarterly Journal of Studies on Alcohol*, **35**, 841–55.

O'Malley, S. S., Jaffe, A. J., Change, G., Schottenfeld, R. S., Meyer, R. E. and Rounsaville, B. (1992) Naltexone and coping skills therapy for alcohol dependence. *Archives of General Psychiatry*, **49**, 881–7.

Oppenheimer, E., Tobutt, C., Taylor, C. and Andrew, T. (1994) Death and survival in a cohort of heroin addicts from London clinics: a 22 year follow-up study. *Addiction*, **89**, 1299–308.

Rollnick, S., Kinnersley, P. and Stott, N. (1993) Methods of helping patients with behaviour change. *British Medical Journal*, **307**, 188–90.

Rosenow, D. J., Niaura, R. S., Childress, A. R., Abrams, D. B. and Monti, P. M. (1991) Cue reactivity in addictive behaviours: theoretical and treatment implications. *International Journal of the Addictions*, **25**, 957–93.

Rossow, I. (1994) Suicide among drug addicts in Norway. *Addiction*, **89**, 1667–73.

Saunders, J. B. (1989) The efficacy of treatment for drinking problems. *International Review of Psychiatry*, **1**, 121–38.

Sisson, R. W. and Azrin, N. H. (1989) The community reinforcement approach. In: Hester, R. and Miller, W. R. (eds.) *Handbook of Alcoholism Treatment Approaches*, pp. 242–58. New York: Pergamon.

Stapleton, J. A., Russell, M. A. H., Feyerabend, C. *et al.* (1995) Dose effects and predictors of outcome in a randomized trial of transdermal nicotine patches in general practice. *Addiction*, **90**, 31–42.

Thom, B., Brown, C., Drummond, C., Edwards, G., Mullan, M. and Taylor C. (1992) Engaging patients with alcohol problems in treatment: the first consultation. *British Journal of Addiction*, **87**, 601–11.

Vaillant, G. E. (1973) A 20-year follow-up of New York narcotic addicts. *Archives of General Psychiatry*, **29**, 237–41.

Vaillant, G. E. (1981) Dangers of psychotherapy in the treatment of alcoholism. In: Bean, M. H. and Zimberg, N. E. (eds.) *Dynamic Approaches to the Understanding and Treatment of Alcoholism*, pp. 36–54. New York: Free Press.

Vaillant, G. E. (1983) *The Natural History of Alcoholism*. Cambridge: Harvard University Press.

Woody, G. E., Luborsky, L., McLellan, A. T. *et al.* (1983) Psychotherapy for opiate addicts. Does it help? *Archives of General Psychiatry*, **40**, 639–45.

Woody, G. E., McLellan, A. T., Luborsky, L. and O'Brien, C. P. (1987) Twelve month follow-up of psychotherapy for opiate dependence. *American Journal of Psychiatry*, **144**, 590–6.

Zimberg, S. (1985) Principles of alcoholism psychotherapy. In: Zimberg, S., Wallace, J. and Blume, S. B. (eds.) *Practical Approaches to Alcoholism Psychotherapy*, 2nd edn., pp. 3–22. New York: Plenum.

7

Advances in families and couples therapy

K. EIA ASEN

The development of systemic family therapy

The field of family and couple therapy has seen many changes over the past four decades. With its roots in family interaction research, systemic family therapy now blossoms in many different contexts, ranging from specialised clinics to psychiatric hospitals, schools, social services and commercial organisations. Whether the term 'advances', with its connotation of progress, is justified, is ultimately for the reader to decide. Some of the changes could be viewed as leaps forward, others perhaps more like two steps backward. And there are those old and familiar practices that are described in trendy terminology – which is about the only thing that is new about them.

Perhaps the most significant impetus for the development of family therapy came from a group of researchers and clinicians in Palo Alto, led by the anthropologist Gregory Bateson. They were particularly interested in studying the patterns of schizophrenic transaction. The group analysed schizophrenic communication and postulated that it was the family of the schizophrenic that had shaped their thought processes via the often bizarre communication requirements imposed on them (Bateson et al. 1956; Bateson, 1978). Bateson and his co-workers also observed that frequently, when the patient got better, someone else in the family appeared to get worse. At times it seemed that the family required a symptomatic person so that it could function better. In fact, the symptomatic person, or 'identified patient' appeared to get stuck in that role and it could then be noticed that everyone resisted change – even if that meant resisting or blocking the clinical improvement of the identified patient. Jackson (1957) termed this phenomenon 'family homeostasis' and viewed the family as a 'system' with equilibrium-maintaining properties, such as coalitions, covert conflicts and scapegoatism. Jackson and other members of Bateson's original group then widened their interests to a whole range of families, not just those containing a schizophrenic member (Watzlawick *et al.*, 1967), in an attempt to classify 'typical' communication and interaction patterns over this broad range of families. Interestingly, in Britain the work of Laing and Esterson (1971) initially also focused on the families of patients diagnosed as suffering from schizophrenia. They came up with similar findings to those of Bateson's early study group: they argued that confusing and mystified communication patterns inside the family led to the ill person's distorted perceptions.

The development of new treatment methods involving the whole family went hand in hand with the academic study of family phenomenology and communication patterns. As psychodynamic thinking constituted a major ethos prevailing in the 1950s and 60s, many of the pioneers in the field of family therapy happened to have been trained as psychoanalysts or psychotherapists. The work of Ackerman (1966) was influential in trying to combine psychoanalytic and family systems ideas and practices. Over the following decades one can observe how psychoanalytic ideas were relinquished and how family therapy has tended to become synonymous with the term 'systems approach'. Its practitioners have adopted the idea of the family as an open system (von Bertalanffy, 1968), with the individual family members being the elements interacting with one another. In doing so, family therapists were initially deliberately uninterested in discovering the reasons as to why individuals were feeling or doing what they felt or did. After all, people were seen as being part of a larger system and behaved according to a set of explicit or implicit rules. Consequently, there was much preoccupation with the how of interaction, and a special focus on observable behaviours of family members in sessions. Looking back it seems that this turning-away from psychoanalytic theory and method may have been a necessary developmental phase for the family therapy movement to have gone through, since it enabled therapists to find radical new ways of practising without being weighed down by traditional psychodynamic concepts. It is only more recently that some of the latter are being 'rediscovered', and integrated into the systemic therapies (Dare, 1988).

Family therapy has broken many taboos before coming of age, and perhaps more than anything it was the new technologies that heralded the advent of a new age of psychotherapy. Hoffman (1981) made the point that the arrival of the one-way screen, which clinicians and researchers have used to observe live family sessions, has been as significant as the invention of the telescope. Viewing the world differently makes it possible to think innovatively. Videotaping family sessions and studying them afterwards allows the therapist to see things from a different perspective. New perspectives produced major discoveries as to how interactions were inter-linked and could be understood in more than one way. Replaying the same videotape of a specific family interaction over and over, with the possibility of pausing and using slow motion, allowed family therapists to study sequences in minute detail. This made it possible to look at what preceded a specific behaviour or communication, how this affected other people in the room, and how the reaction, in turn, affected further communications. Problem behaviours seemed clearly interlinked, as it was often impossible to determine what came first, the chicken or the egg. Such recursive processes are described by the term 'circularity', where communication 'a' leads to communication 'b',which leads to communication 'c', which in turn leads to more of communication 'a', and so on. When these loops repeat themselves frequently we use the notion of 'pattern'. For instance, in this classic example:

He: 'I only drink because you upset me.'
She: 'But I am only upset because you drink.'
He: 'If you weren't upsetting me all the time I would stop drinking . . .'
She: 'If you stopped drinking I wouldn't be upset.'

each partner views his or her actions merely as a reaction to the other's behaviours. It is left to an outside observer to point out the circularity of their interaction, namely that the husband's drinking elicits the wife's behaviour which, in turn, elicits his drinking, which elicits her being upset, which . . . and so on. Family therapy aims to challenge and disrupt such dysfunctional patterns so that new forms of communication and interaction can emerge. This has produced a whole range of family therapy models and strategies of which the four most influential are described in the following section.

The structural approach

Structural family therapy was developed by Minuchin and co-workers (Minuchin et al., 1967; Minuchin, 1974), and many of its ideas are based on a normative model of family functioning. This model holds that family structure becomes 'visible' through the ways the various subsystems such as children, parents and grandparents interact, and how the boundaries are negotiated between them. It is assumed that families function particularly well when semi-permeable boundaries are in existence, for instance around the partners to protect their privacy, between the parents and the children to allow a hierarchical system with sufficient flow of information up and down, or around the nuclear family so that it can preserve its identity and rules whilst at the same time being receptive to the outside world.

The therapist's task is to intervene in such a way as to make the family structure approximate this normative model. Techniques include challenging directly absent or rigid boundaries, 'unbalancing' the family equilibrium by temporarily joining with one member of the family against others, or setting 'homework' tasks designed to restore hierarchies. The structural approach is very active, with the therapist encouraging family members to 'enact' problems in the consulting room so that the ways in which communications become blocked or interactions get entrenched can be studied. One fairly dramatic technique designed to achieve this is 'intensification', whereby the therapist deliberately increases the tension in the room and lets family members go beyond their normal limits in the hope that this will induce a therapeutic crisis, and result in the family discovering new resources and solutions.

Not surprisingly, the structural approach has attracted a lot of criticism, attractive though it is to the beginner as providing clear guidelines for the therapist. The most common accusations are that it is not only a form of social engineering, but also culturally insensitive and 'male'. These criticisms have resulted in a considerable change in the practice of structural therapy in recent years. Instead of the therapist defining for the family what would be best for them, he or she elicits from them their blueprint of family functioning, one that fits the family's prevailing beliefs and its cultural setting. Once the family has defined its goals it becomes the therapist's task to help the family to achieve these. This helps the therapist to respect the norms of different cultures and sub-cultures. A number of practitioners (Goodrich, 1991; Vetere, 1993) have shown that the model can be modified to be gender sensitive.

Strategic and Brief Therapy approaches

The term 'strategic' (Haley, 1963) describes any therapy in which the clinician actively designs interventions or 'strategies' to fit the problem (Hoffman, 1981). Therapy initially does not appear to focus on the family as a whole but rather narrowly on the details of the presenting symptom. The underlying assumption is that the symptom is being maintained by the apparent 'solution' – the very behaviours that seek to suppress it. For example, the 'shy' adolescent may elicit parental over-protectiveness, a solution that may well perpetuate the problem. A structural therapist might be inclined to view over-protectiveness as part of the family organisation, linked to past family scripts or myths, and therefore challenge communication patterns that may be indirectly linked to the presenting problem. Strategic therapists, on the other hand, would not concern themselves with other dysfunctional behaviours unless these are presented as problems. Instead, they focus on the problem brought by the client or family in an attempt to solve it (Watzlawick *et al.*, 1974; Haley, 1977). It could be argued that this is nevertheless systemic work, because if one thing changes then a domino effect can be observed in other interactions and behaviours as well.

Strategic therapists use 'reframing' as a major technique. The family or client's perceived problem(s) are put into a different meaning-frame that provides new perspectives and therefore makes new behaviours possible. An example is the salesman who wanted help for his stammer and was told by the strategic therapist that this was not a defect but an asset since people were more likely to pay attention to someone who had trouble talking. He was encouraged to increase his stammering in order to become a more successful salesman (Watzlawick *et al.*, 1974). Such positive reframing with the simultaneous prescription of the symptom seems bizarre to many mental health professionals, and has earned some strategic therapists the reputation of being manipulative or making fun of their patients' suffering. Unfortunately, some such 'clever' interventions have distracted from the many useful ideas contained in this approach. Like behaviour therapy, it has a narrow focus and deals in the first instance with the problem, and is therefore acceptable to families and individuals as it does not implicitly hold the family responsible. It often prepares the ground for further work as other family issues gradually emerge. The strategic therapies are primarily symptomatic approaches and therapy is usually not a long-term enterprise. In fact, the fashionable term 'Brief Therapy' is frequently used when referring to certain strategic approaches. One of these and a more recent development is Michael White's work (White, 1989), which attempts to externalise the symptom. For example, an encopretic child is encouraged to think of the soiling as his enemy, 'sneaky pooh', who needs to be defeated. The help of the family is enlisted to devise strategies to trick this imaginary monster. Soon all forces are joined to outwit the symptom, which becomes the enemy of the whole family, and this playful approach is particularly popular with families with young children.

A phenomenon of the 90s is the rapid growth of 'solution focused' therapies, in parallel with dominant political ideologies that do not wish to examine the causes of illness and dysfunction, but instead look at solutions. De Shazer's (1985) work has found many followers, partly because of its pragmatism, partly because it is a method that is rapidly learned and appears to yield fast results. De Shazer observed that symptoms and problems have a tendency to fluctuate. A depressed person, for example, is sometimes more and sometimes less depressed. Focusing on the times when he or she is less depressed, the exceptions are identified on which therapeutic strategies are built. These exceptions form the basis of the solution. If clients are encouraged to amplify the 'solution' patterns of behaviours, then the problem patterns can be driven into the background (George *et al.*, 1990).

Milan systemic approaches

The work of the original Milan team (Selvini Palazzoli *et al.*, 1978) has undergone considerable changes over the past 15 years. The group initially involved itself in research on families with anorexic and schizophrenic members. Based on Bateson's (Bateson *et al.*, 1956) and the Palo Alto group's work (Watzlawick *et al.*, 1967), the Milan team developed a theory about 'family games' and strategies for changing the rules of these games. In marked contrast to the 'Brief Therapies', the Milan team had considerable interest in multi-generational family patterning, and ways of describing the interactions and struggles of family members over several generations (Jones, 1993). This involved making elaborate hypotheses about how, for instance, a young adult might have got caught up in his parents' seemingly endless conflicts. In such a case it can be surmised that each parent disqualifies the other with pressure on the young adult to take a position to support either mother or father. Unwilling to take sides and thereby risking alienation of a parent, he may feel trapped and it could be hypothesised that his 'solution' to this dilemma is to opt out and act 'mad'. Such hypotheses led to the design of interventions that took into account the anticipated attempts of the family to disqualify the therapy. The resulting 'counter-paradoxes' prescribed by the Milan team were aimed at recommending 'no change' in the hope that the family would resist this command and do the opposite, namely change – if only to defeat the therapists.

In order to confirm or refute hypotheses about family process and to arrive at these interventions, the Milan team perfected a particular interviewing technique: circular questioning (Selvini Palzzoli *et al.*, 1980). The therapist conducts the family session mostly by asking questions, seeking information about people, their differences and the various relationships and their specific characteristics. Such questions might, for instance, be triadic in that they ask person A about his perception of aspects of the relationship between persons B and C. Talking about this in the presence of everyone inevitably produces feedback from everyone, feedback on which the therapist bases his next questions. By responding to feedback from the individual family members the therapist enacts the systemic notion of the circularity of interaction.

In the early 1980s the Milan group divided into two groups, with Selvini Palazzoli *et al.* (1989) pursuing her interests in unravelling the 'games' of psychotic and anorexic families. She became increasingly preoccupied with designing an 'invariate' prescription, a specific intervention she believed should be given to all families after a few sessions. This intervention, which prescribes mysterious parental disappearance acts, aims at disrupting 'chronic' family organisation and thereby temporarily creating a stronger boundary between the parental generation and their adult children, a move not unlike certain structural techniques. Palazzoli observed that this intervention, effective though it seemed in many cases, appeared to have little effect in quite a few others. This finding led her group to rethink the wisdom of the same prescription being given to every family irrespective of their presenting problems.

The other half of the original Milan team (Boscolo *et al.*, 1987) went in the opposite direction, away from any prescriptiveness, to what was later termed a 'co-constructivist approach'. This has now given way to the term 'post-Milan', in line with the current vogue for anything not so new being disguised with the prefix 'post-'. What this group and their numerous followers are concerned with is the critique of objectivity, namely the traditional scientific view that the observer (or clinician) stands outside the process observed. Inspired by the writings of physicists, neuroscientists and philosophers (Maturana and Varela, 1972; Capra, 1975; von Foerster, 1981) the post-Milan therapists focus on how the observer actually constructs that which is being observed. They developed new interviewing techniques, fashionably called 'conversations', whereby family and therapist 'co-evolve' or 'co-construct' new ways of describing the family system in such a way that it no longer needs to be viewed or experienced as problematic (Jones, 1993). The characteristics of a post-Milan therapist are those of a clinician who is 'democratic' and realistic about the possibility of change, with no wish to impose personal ideas, being alert to openings and curious about his or her own position in the observed system, taking non-judgmental and multi-positional stances.

Behavioural family therapy approaches

Among the more recent arrivals on the family therapy scene are the behavioural family therapists. The interventions are derived from the principles of social learning theory (Jacobson and Margolin, 1979). Treatment starts with a behavioural analysis and aims to pinpoint specific family problems and goals. Intervention strategies include, amongst others, communication training, contingency contracting, problem-solving training, limit setting, operant-conditioning strategies and, as in other brands of family therapy, homework tasks (Falloon, 1988). The modern behavioural family therapist gets the family to decide which specific problems are to be addressed. The focus is on searching for creative solutions from within the family, with the therapist in the role of a facilitator rather than an expert problem-solver.

The psycho-educational approach (Leff *et al.*, 1982; Anderson, 1983) has strong behavioural elements though it also draws from structural techniques. It is based on the findings that schizophrenics who return to live with a family whose attitudes towards the ill person are critical or emotionally over-involved (high Expressed Emotion or EE), are significantly more likely to relapse in the nine months following discharge from hospital than those patients who return to low EE families. Consequently, the aim of therapy is to reduce the emotional intensity as well as the degree of physical proximity. This is achieved by three separate therapeutic ingredients: educational sessions for the family, about schizophrenia and the part the family can play in keeping the patient well; a fortnightly relatives' group, to share experiences and solutions; and family sessions (Kuipers *et al.*, 1992).

The coming of age of family and couple therapy

The terms and terminology of family therapy and the concepts they describe have more recently come under scrutiny. Jones (1993) points out that the term 'family' is often read as implying an intact, two-parent, heterosexual couple with about two children and two pets, with the man the breadwinner and woman the homemaker. At a time when the traditional nuclear family is in decline such a picture is hardly any longer the norm and risks pathologising other family forms such as gay or lesbian couples, single parents with children, childless couples and unattached adults. Nowadays, multiple forms of committed relationships coexist in our cultures which makes the term 'family therapy' seem increasingly a misnomer. It is not necessary to have a family in order to work with family therapy ideas: any relationship lends itself to this, hence the emergence of the new terms 'systems therapists' or 'relationship therapist'.

Moreover, the term 'therapy' itself can imply illness and dysfunction that require cures. In fact, there are plenty of families who regard it as outrageous that they should be thought of as being in need of therapy, with the suggestion that there is something wrong with them or that they are the cause of one of their member's pathology. Many practitioners now tend to use more neutral words to describe their activity, such as 'family meetings' or 'family consultation',

Some family therapists (see, for instance, Whitaker, 1982) insist that the 'whole family' (therapist's definition) should attend. For some therapists this may well require the attendance not only of the nuclear family but also of all grandparents, uncles and aunts. If any of them cannot or will not make it, the session is cancelled. Needless to say, such practices are now rare as the cancellation rates with this model are very high, and purchasers of health care are unlikely to tolerate and fund such ventures. In general, many family therapists nowadays will invite 'the family' for the first session, but see whoever turns up. It is not uncommon for the number of clients attending the actual therapy sessions to increase over time from one person to as many as six or ten, including members of the extended family or relevant others, so long as it is made clear that the 'therapeutic system' is open, and ready for others to join if and when it seems right for them (Jenkins and Asen, 1992).

A few words should be said at this point about the differences between family and couple therapy. If one subscribes to the model of an open therapeutic system, then what may start as 'couple therapy' may sooner or later include children or in-laws. Similarly, many family therapies may develop into couple therapies when it makes sense to family and therapist to concentrate on issues between partners. However, some of the demands made upon the therapist during couple sessions are different from family work and deserve a mention. With two partners present the therapist becomes the third person, with pressure on him or her to act as arbitrator with an open almost irresistible 'pull' to take sides. The gender of the therapist may evoke fears in a client of not getting a fair hearing, because the therapist is seen as having the 'wrong' gender or the 'wrong ' sexual orientation. Moreover, feelings of rivalry or contempt may be stirred up. A willingness on the part of the therapist to address these issues openly is an important therapeutic stance.

Family therapists, perhaps more than any other group of mental health professionals, have in recent years become increasingly preoccupied with gender, race and class issues, and how these affect clinical practice. Since the systemic therapies are concerned with viewing people and their presenting problems in multiple contexts, this is not a development that is surprising: gender assumptions, racism, and class prejudice are all-powerful determinants of behaviour. Many family therapists have started examining their own professional attitudes in relation to these issues and more sensitive and appropriate practices are developing (Goldner, 1991; Boyd-Franklin, 1989), both when consulting with individual clients or families, as well as when dealing with the larger professional networks.

Whilst family and couple therapy continues to grow in the USA mostly in private practice, in Britain many professionals work with the systemic model in primary care and specialist settings, ranging from health visitors and GPs to teachers, social workers, nurses, psychologists, psychiatrists and others. In addition, one now also finds specialist jobs advertised specifically for 'family therapists'. Has family therapy then become a treatment modality that is best dispensed by trained specialist family therapists? It is important to make the distinction between family therapy as one of a number of psychological treatment methods and family therapy as a way of conceptualising psychological and psychosocial disturbance. The latter, namely the ability to think in terms of systems, is an indispensable tool for any clinician as it helps to view the patient, the family, and the institution in context, and informs the clinical management. Subsequently the application of systemic ideas and practices to quite diverse work contexts is only a natural development. The practice of family therapy is no longer confined to special rooms equipped with one-way mirrors, videos, microphones, and teams of four. Family therapy has moved from its elitist stance and become user-friendly (Treacher and Carpenter, 1993). Systemic work is now done in such diverse settings as mediation services (Robinson, 1991), general practice (Asen and Tomson, 1992), paediatrics (Minuchin *et al.*, 1978; Lask, 1982), oncology units (Wellfish and Cohen, 1986) and schools (Dowling and Osborne, 1985; Dawson and McHugh, 1994) – to mention but a few. Multi-family group work is gaining more impetus, particularly in the field of child abuse and neglect (Asen *et al.*, 1989), and increasingly work takes place in people's homes and community settings (Clark *et al.*, 1982).

Integrating family therapy approaches

The field of family therapy is flourishing. Different models are in operation and whilst there are those practitioners who adhere to one particular
school with missionary zeal, the majority of family therapists have found
their own blend, drawing on a whole range of different ideas and practices. Clearly, family therapy models and interventions need to be
matched to agency contexts: what may work in a specialised family therapy is seen as a mere adjunct to biological treatments. Family therapist
purists are irritating to those having to work with them as they see
themselves not only as 'meta' to the professional system of which they
themselves are part, but also 'better' than their allegedly unenlightened
colleagues. Cecchin *et al.* (1992) remind us that a healthy irreverence
towards one's own ideas is a necessity for any therapist to ensure flexibility and creativity. Once therapists fall in love with their models and
believe these to be true and universal, complexity will be reduced to some
banal principles, with 'invariate' prescriptions or other entirely predictable interventions levelled at anyone, irrespective of their personal characteristics or family circumstances. Whilst such a stance may be
reassuring to the therapist it probably is of rather limited value to clients
and their families.

Does family therapy work? There are now a considerable number of
family therapy outcome studies (see, for example, Leff *et al.*, 1982;
Russell *et al.*, 1987), which demonstrate its efficacy. Many of these and
other studies are, however, criticised on methodological grounds. So far
very few attempts have been made to provide family therapy treatment
manuals that clearly describe the methods used. Predictably, many family
therapists argue that any manualised treatment goes against the notion of
therapy, which is meant to be a spontaneous, flexible and creative process. Moreover, they criticise conventional research methods and outcome criteria as not fitting the systemic epistemology (Asen *et al.*,
1991). Despite many reservations, more and more family therapists are
involving themselves in researching and evaluating the outcome of their
work. These ventures, together with the continued development of their
specific theoretical concepts and clinical skills, allow family therapists to
contribute significantly to the understanding and management of psychosocial disorders.

References

Ackerman, N. W. (1966) *Treating the Troubled Family*. New York: Basic Books.

Anderson, C. M. (1983) A psychoeducational program for families of patients with schizophrenia. In: McFarlane, W. (ed.) *Family Therapy in Schizophrenia*, pp. 99–116. New York: Guilford Press.

Asen, K., Berkowitz, R., Cooklin, A., Leff, J., Piper, R. and Rein, L. (1991) Family therapy outcome research: a trial for families, therapists and researchers. *Family Process*, **30**, 3–20.

Asen, K., George, E., Piper, R. and Stevens, A. (1989) A systems approach to child abuse: management and treatment issues. *Child Abuse and Neglect*, **13**, 45–57.

Asen, K. E. and Tomson, P. (1992) *Family Solutions in Family Practice*. Lancaster: Quay Publishing.

Bateson, G. (1978) The birth of a matrix or double blind and epistemology. In: Berger, M. (ed.) *Beyond the Double Bind*, pp. 39–64. New York: Bruner/Mazel.

Bateson, G., Jackson, D., Haley, J. and Weakland, J. (1956) Toward a theory of schizophrenia. *Behavioural Science*, **1**, 251–64.

Boscolo, L., Cecchin, G., Hoffman, L. and Penn, P. (1987) *Milan Systemic Family Therapy*. New York: Basic Books.

Boyd-Franklin, N. (1989) *Black Families in Therapy: A Multisystems Approach*. New York: Guilford Press.

Capra, F. (1975) *The Tao of Physics*. London: Fontana/Collins.

Cecchin, G., Lane, G. and Ray, W. A. (1992) *Irreverence: A Strategy for Therapists' Survival*. London: Karnac Books.

Clark, T., Zalis, T. and Sacco, F. (1982) *Outreach Family Therapy*. New York: J. Aronson.

Dare, C. (1988) Psychoanalytic family therapy. In: Street, E. and Dryden, W. (eds.) *Family Therapy in Britain*, pp. 23–50. Milton Keynes: Open University Press.

Dawson, N. and McHugh, B. (1994) Parents and children: Participants in change. In: Dowling, E. and Osborne, E. (eds.) *The Family and the School* (2nd edn), pp. 81–101. London: Routledge and Kegan Paul.

de Shazer, S. (1985) *Keys to Solutions in Brief Therapy*. New York: W. W. Norton.

Dowling, E. and Osborne, E. (eds.) (1985) *The Family and the School. A Joint Systems Approach to Problems with Children*. London: Routledge and Kegan Paul.

Falloon, I. R. H. (1988) Behavioural systems therapy: systems, structures and strategies. In: Street, E. and Dryden, W. (eds.) *Family Therapy in Britain*, pp. 101–26. Milton Keynes: Open University Press.

George, E., Iveson, C. and Ratner, H. (1990 *Problem to Solution*. London: Brief Therapy Press.

Goldner, V. (1991) Feminism and systemic practice: two critical traditions in transition. *Journal of Family Therapy*, **13**, 95–104.

Goodrich, T. D. (1991) *Women and Power: Perspective for Family Therapy*. New York: W. W. Norton & Co.

Haley, J. (1963) *Strategies of Psychotherapy*. New York: Grune and Stratton.

Haley, J. (1977) *Problem-solving Therapy*. San Francisco, Jossey-Bass.

Hoffmann, L. (1981) *Foundations of Family Therapy*. New York: Basic Books.

Jackson, D. (1957) The question of family homeostasis. *Psychiatric Quarterly Supplement*, **31**, 79–90.

Jacobson, N. S. and Margolin, G. (1979) *Marital Therapy: Strategies Based on Social Learning and Behavior Exchanges Principles*. New York: Brunner/ Mazel.

Jenkins, H. and Asen, K. (1992) Family therapy without the family: a framework for systemic practice. *Journal of Family Therapy*, **14**, 1–14.

Jones, E. (1993) *Family Systems Therapy*. Chichester/New York: John Wiley & Son.

Kuipers, L., Leff, J. and Lam. D. (1992) *Family Work for Schizophrenia: A Practical Guide*. London: Gaskell.

Laing, R. D. and Esterson, A. (1971) *Sanity, Madness and the Family*. New York; Basic Books.

Lask, B. (1982) Family therapy in a paediatric setting. In: Bentovim, A., Gorell Barnes, G. and Cooklin, A. (eds.) *Family Therapy: Complimentary Frameworks of Theory and Practice*, pp. 465–78. London: Academic Press.

Leff, J., Kuipers, L., Berkowitz, R., Eberlein-Vries, R. and Sturgeon, D. (1982) A controlled trial of social intervention in the families of schizophrenic patients. *British Journal of Psychiatry*, **141**, 121–34.

Maturana, H. R. and Varela, F. J. (1972) *Autopoiesis and Cognition: The Realization of Living*. Dordrecht: Reidel Public.

Minuchin, S. (1974) *Families and Family Therapy*. London: Tavistock.

Minuchin, S., Montalvo, B., Guerney, B. G., Rosman, B. L. and Schumer, F. (1967) *Families of the Slums*. New York: Basic Books.

Minuchin, S., Rosman, B. L. and Baker, L. (1978) *Psychosomatic Families*. Cambridge Mass.: Harvard University Press.

Robinson, M. (1991) *Family Transfomation Through Divorce and Remarriage: A Systemic Approach*. London: Routledge.

Russell, G. F., Szmukler, G. I. and Dare, C. (1987) An evaluation of family therapy in anorexia nervosa and bulimia nervosa. *Archives of General Psychiatry*, **44**, 1047–56.

Selvini Palazzoli, M., Boscolo, L., Cecchin, L. and Prata, G. (1978) *Paradox and Counterparadox*. New York: J. Aronson.

Selvini Palazzoli, M., Boscolo, L., Cecchin, G. and Prata, G. (1980) Hypothesizing, circularity, neutrality: three guidelines for the conductor of the session. *Family Process*, **19**, 3–12.

Selvini Palazzoli, M., Cirillo, S., Selvini, M. and Sorrentino, A. M. (1989) *Family Games*. London: Karnac Books.

Treacher, A. and Carpenter, J. (1993) User-friendly family therapy. In: Carpenter, J. and Treacher, A. (eds.) *Using Family Therapy in the 90s*, pp. 8–31. Oxford: Blackwell.

Vetere, A. (1993) Using family therapy in services for people with learning disabilities. In: Carpenter, J. and Treacher, A. (eds.) *Using Family Therapy in the 90s*, pp. 111–30. Oxford: Blackwell.

von Bertalanffy, L. (1968) *General Systems Theory: Foundations, Development Applications*. Harmondsworth: Penguin Books.

von Foerster, H. (1981) *Observing Systems*. Seaside, CA: Intersystems.

Watzlawick, P., Jackson, D. and Beavin, J. (1967) *Pragmatics of Human Communication*. New York: W. W. Norton.

Watzlawick, P., Weakland, J. and Fish, R. (1974) *Change: Principles of Problem Formation and Problem Resolution*. New York: W. W. Norton.

Wellfish, D. K. and Cohen, M. M. (1986) The family therapist as system consultant to medical oncology. In: Wynne, L. C., McDaniel, S. and Weber, T. T. (eds) *Systems Consultation*, pp. 199–218. New York: Guilford Press.

Whitaker, C. (ed. Neill, J. R. and Kniskern, D. P.) (1982) *From Psyche to System*. New York: Guilford Press.

White, M. (1989) *Selected Papers*. Adelaide: Dulwich Centre Publication.

8

Solution focused brief therapy: a co-operative approach to work with clients

HARVEY RATNER AND DENIS YANDOLI

Introduction

In the early 1980s a team of therapists and researchers at the Brief Family Therapy Center in Milwaukee began exploring a new direction in brief therapy. What they discovered is best summed up in a statement from an early article: 'Effective therapy can be done even when the therapist cannot describe what the client is complaining about. Basically, all the therapist and client need to know is "how will we know when the problem is solved?" ' (de Shazer *et al.*, 1986).

The tradition of brief therapy to which the Milwaukee group belonged was that of the Brief Therapy Center at the Mental Research Institute in Palo Alto (Watzlawick *et al.*, 1974). This earlier approach had pioneered a here and now approach to problem solving, based on the notion that 'the attempted solution is the problem', in which it is assumed that problems arise when clients' attempts to deal with everyday difficulties are unsuccessful but are nevertheless repeated in the vain hope of change occurring. For example, a person may be complaining about his or her partner's drinking, which leads to heavier drinking, which leads to more complaining, which leads . . . This approach is non-normative, in the sense that no attempt is made to categorise any person's behaviour as pathological. However, there is an emphasis on exploring what the clients have been doing to solve their problems, and for the therapist to design an intervention to help them do something different. It therefore came as something of a bombshell when Steve de Shazer and his team came upon the idea that to solve a problem it isn't even necessary to know what the problem is – and therefore, this is an approach that can be applied to a wide range of problem presentations.

In this chapter we will describe the solution focused approach, and illustrate the ideas with reference to a clinical case. In keeping with the apparent transferability of this approach from problem to problem, we have not found it useful to make distinctions in the way we work with different substance usage. While clients experience their drug and alcohol usage in different ways, we have found that the approach to helping clients overcome their problems is essentially the same no matter what substance is being misused.

The authors have been developing the application of the approach to drug and alcohol users at the Drug Dependency Unit, St. Mary's Hospital, London for the last five years. In addition, one of the authors (H.R.) has been a member of a brief therapy project in a community mental health clinic, which has published the first British texts on the use of the approach (George *et al.*, 1990).

A competency-based approach: the importance of exceptions to the problem

As an approach that does not think about clients' problems in terms of pathology, but rather as failed attempts to solve difficulties, it follows that the basic philosophy behind brief therapy is the view that clients have the skills and resources necessary to solve their problems. A major contribution of the solution focused approach is that the therapy is focused on the times the problem is less or even non-existent. Clients will usually describe their problems in terms of something happening all the time: they will use the word *always* when talking about the hold the problem has over them: 'Once I've had one pint I always go on to drink eight'; 'Whenever I see X (the supplier) in the street, I always end up getting some gear off him'. Following in de Shazer's footsteps, we find it useful to think that nothing *always* happens and to help the client to think of *exceptions* that, rather than proving the rule that the problem always happens, are evidence that the client has got what it takes to solve his or her problems. This shifts the direction of the whole conversation with the client. Instead of last Wednesday, when the client stopped at three beers rather than going on to eight being seen as a mere fluke, it becomes instead the main focus of discussion between client and therapist. The exception, the time the problem isn't happening or at least is less, can be seen as an indication of the solution in action and a sign of what is working and therefore of what the client needs to do more. In this approach, therefore, less emphasis is placed on understanding how the client's problems have arisen; instead, it is assumed that clients have lost sight of their own abilities and resources. Clients often participate in the social and medical definition of themselves as alcoholics and addicts, labels that narrow the possibilities for change. We see the endeavour of therapy as principally being that of helping clients to see themselves in a different light, one that opens possibilities for change.

The process whereby clients come to see themselves as 'addicts' may have taken place over a long period of time, and frequently they will say that the label has been helpful to them, for example, 'since the doctor told me I was an alcoholic I've realised what a serious problem I have'. Finding an exception to the drinking pattern is of itself not usually going to be enough for clients to change their behaviour. Clients will often need to see and experience the exceptions in their lives in greater detail. Encouraging clients to follow through on tasks has often been seen as a particular difficulty in the field of drug and alcohol misuse, and brief therapists have sought to develop tasks that will be most easily used by clients. If clients perceive the exception as being something that they have some control over and which therefore they can repeat, then they are encouraged 'to do more of what works'. If they are unsure of how to repeat the experience (the situation for the majority of clients), then they are asked to follow one of a number of simple observation tasks.

Steps in the therapy

There are a number of clear steps that can be taken in a solution focused interview. As in other brief therapy approaches, it is usually the first session in which the steps can be most clearly seen:

1. Problem-free talk to build rapport with the client, and problem definition.
2. Establishment of goals for the therapy.
3. Search for exceptions.
4. Ending, consisting of a consultation break, and the delivery of a message to the client.

Problem-free talk and problem definition

When beginning work with a new client it is, of course, necessary to try to develop some rapport with the client. In most approaches it is assumed that the therapist will quickly 'get down to business' and ask questions about the problem, and this is what most clients will also expect. However, this might give the client the message that the therapist believes that it is necessary to talk about and understand the problem in order to solve it, as in other approaches. It would also collude with the view that the client and others may have that the problem is overwhelming, that the client *is* the problem. By beginning instead with a brief conversation about the client's interests, for example, the message can be conveyed to the client that we regard him or her as being more than the problem – that we are interested in him or her as a person and not as a walking problem. The actual problem may then be discussed in as brief a way as possible.

Knowing when the problem is solved: the establishment of goals

Goal definition with clients is a long-established practice in therapy and has become an essential feature of solution focused work. Once the therapist has heard the essential detail of the problem, he or she will wish to move as quickly as possible to an examination of what the client would like to see happening in his or her life once that problem is solved. Once the client has defined how he or she will know that drinking, for example, is no longer a problem, then locating exceptions to his or her drinking behaviour (i.e. times when he or she is already drinking less) will make an enormous difference in motivation to institute change-making behaviours. Without a sense of where the client wants to get to, there is going to be much less hope about actually moving forward. Once a goal is identified, an expectation of change begins to grow, especially if the goal is seen as small and salient to the client.

There are a number of characteristics of workable goals that it is important to aim for, including that they should be described in as concrete and specific behavioural detail as possible. One of the most important features (de Shazer, 1991) is that the goal should describe the *start* of something and not the end. Clients typically are very good at describing what they do not want to see happening in their lives, such as, 'I won't be drinking so heavily', 'I won't be so depressed', 'he won't be spending all our money on drugs'. However, the absence of something cannot constitute a goal to be aimed for: the goal needs to be stated in terms of what will be happening *instead* of the problem behaviour. We often find ourselves asking clients questions such as, 'so when that is no longer a problem to you, what will be happening instead?' 'What will you see him doing instead that will tell you he is controlling his drinking?'

Perhaps the most well-known intervention designed by de Shazer and his colleagues is the so-called 'Miracle question' (de Shazer, 1988), which acts as a particularly useful goals-focused question:

Imagine that tonight, while you are asleep, a miracle happens, and the problem that brought you here is solved. Because you are asleep you don't know the miracle has happened, but when you wake up you begin to do things that tell you a miracle has happened. What will be the first thing you will start to do? And the next . . . ? What will your partner notice you doing that will tell them that a miracle has happened?

In our experience, the idea of a miracle helps clients to make a mental leap away from the present time and their oppressive problems in the here and now, and to be able to envision how they would like things to be. We have found that two conditions are important as prerequisites to a smooth use of this question, namely that a co-operative relationship has been engendered between therapist and client beforehand, so that clients are ready to take the question seriously, and that the therapist is clear about what it is that the miracle is solving – if one says 'a miracle happens and your life becomes as you want it to be', you cannot be surprised if the client begins talking about a future after winning the lottery! Such an answer is unlikely to help the therapeutic process. In most of our cases we find clients give answers that are realistic and down to earth. The 'other person perspective' questions as above ('What will your partner notice you doing?') are helpful in enabling the client to enlarge his or her miracle picture by drawing in other perspectives, and for looking at changes in relationships that need to occur: 'So when your husband is no longer drinking, what will you be doing then? How will he know you're pleased that he's no longer drinking?'

Connecting the future to the present: the search for exceptions

Although the idea of the exception is the basis of this therapy, the early part of the work is focused on goal clarification. It is a goal-led therapy, so to speak. Once the client has begun defining his or her goals, the therapist can move to asking about the exceptions, which in the context of the goals work already done, can be described as 'signs of the miracle happening'. Indeed, de Shazer has recently proposed (1994) that the term 'exceptions' be replaced by 'hidden miracles'. So the therapist will ask questions to ascertain 'the signs, however small, that tell you the miracle is already starting to happen'. He or she will ask the client to think back to a recent time when things were better or at least not as bad as things currently are, and ask the client to try to expand on what they were doing then to bring the changes about. The client will be invited to consider the perspective of important others in his or her life: what it is that others would say they have seen the client do to help their situation. Wherever possible questions are phrased in a way that shows the therapist's expectation of change: '*When* was the last time you said no to the offer of cocaine' and '*What* did you do on that occasion' is more likely to engage the client in searching for such an occasion than if he or she is asked a more closed question such as '*Has* there been a time . . . '. Each occasion of difference is scrutinised for what it tells client and therapist alike about the client's proven capability in solving the problem.

It is quite rare for a client to insist that there are no times when things have been better. When this happens, however, an important area of exceptions interviewing becomes to find out how the client is *coping* with his or her situation. No matter how bad the situation is, there is something that he or she is doing to keep on going and to stop things from getting even worse, and these things need to be scrutinised as before.

An area of questioning that has taken a prominent place in solution focused interviewing is the use of scale or ratings questions. Clients will be asked to rate their progress towards their goals on a 0 to 10 scale: 'If 0 represents where you were when you were first referred to this clinic, and 10 represents the day after the miracle has happened, where would you say you're at today? What have you done to move from 0 to x (where x represents the client's initial reply)? What would your partner say you have done to move to x? What will you be doing when you have reached $x + ?$'. Scale questions are extraordinarily effective in helping clients to be specific about what they have been doing to get themselves from zero to where they are now (i.e. the exceptions), and to think about what the next small step would be. One of the strengths of these questions is that they help clients who have otherwise been very vague about their goals to nevertheless have a goal to aim for: i.e. it is '10', even if neither client nor therapist has much of an idea what it actually looks like. It is also very useful to ask clients to rate their *confidence* at achieving a certain goal. If a client's confidence of the possibility of change is low then it is important to ascertain what they would need to see that would help their confidence in change to be strengthened.

Feelings in brief therapy

It is clear that there is a strong emphasis in brief therapy on helping clients to describe their goals and their progress in behavioural terms. This, however, is not to discount their emotional life. Clients, obviously, will talk not only about their feelings regarding the problem itself, but also the feelings they hope to have in the wished-for future. It is not, for example, uncommon for someone, having described his or her problem as 'being depressed', to then say that after a miracle he or she would be 'feeling happy' instead. Asked for greater clarification, the reply may be 'I'll just know when I'm feeling happier'. The brief therapist will acknowledge the yearning behind these words, but will gently perservere in attempting to help the client to describe what he or she will be *doing* when happier, as a goal such as 'to feel happy' is too vague to set as a target. Questions such as 'What will your mother see you doing that will tell her you are feeling happy?' are ways to lead towards greater clarity. In some cases it may be necessary to explore the feeling states in greater detail until the client can make a bridge to a behavioural description. For example, 'So, what else will you be feeling when you are feeling happier?' 'Relaxed.' 'OK, so when you are feeling relaxed what else will you be feeling?' 'More confident.' 'And when you are feeling more confident, what will you start to *do* then?' 'I guess I might start looking for a job.'

It is not assumed that the exploration and expression of emotion is of itself important in the resolution of problems. If it is the first time that the client has spoken about certain things (such as bereavement, or experience of childhood abuse) then the client might well find such a conversation to be very helpful, but in general we find that the client needs to talk about his or her feelings and problems generally, only up to the point that he or she feels that the therapist has demonstrated an understanding of the significance of what the client has and is enduring.

It is important to stress here that an approach to therapy that assumes competence in clients will be experienced as insensitive if the therapist is not able to acknowledge the very real and serious impact that poverty, inequality and racism can have on people's lives. These are external, hard facts in clients' lives, and there is no place for a kind of naive optimism that clients can overcome the trials of, say, homelessness without great hardship. As has been indicated earlier, in many situations it is important to ask how clients are able to *cope* with a certain situation. For example, 'While you are waiting for rehousing/a place in a residential unit/for your partner to leave, etc. how are you going to cope? How are you going to look after yourself in such a way that you don't end up drinking and making yourself ill?'

Sometimes the feelings clients have about their situation will influence the course of the interview. Clients who say they don't feel they have a particular problem with drugs, 'It's just that my partner/my probation officer/my doctor, etc. thinks I have', will need to be asked what *they* would find useful in coming to the sessions. As far as possible clients should be helped to establish the goals that they have for treatment. If their aim is considerably at odds with the referrer's expressed goals then a way has to be found to compromise, rather than to impose goals on them. Clients may not feel they use drugs excessively, but would nevertheless be willing to work towards a reduced usage if that would mean, for example, that their partners would complain less to them about their behaviour.

Ending sessions and giving tasks

Just as it is the task of the therapist to explore a client's strengths and resources, so it is essential to give the client positive feedback at all times as to what, in the therapist's opinion, is useful solution-building behaviour and attitudes. Some clients respond with increasing curiosity about the different picture that is emerging about themselves and their strengths. Others are less certain and will 'Yes, but . . . ' the therapist on occasion–which does not mean the therapist should stop complimenting the client. Instead it will be necessary to find a way to feedback to the client that helps him or her to be more receptive, perhaps by being tentative, for example, 'I don't know how significant it is that you stayed away from that place yesterday, but I can see it took some doing'.

In general it is found helpful to give some formal feedback to the client at the end of the session, preferably after the therapist has taken a five-minute 'think' break about 45 minutes into the session. This feedback will compliment the client on the efforts he or she has made to tackle problems, and any other feedback the therapist thinks might be useful to give, such as complimenting the client on having been able to get to the session. The feedback message will then finish with the suggestion of a homework task, and the session (no more than an hour in length) will end once the question of a further session has been explored.

Observation tasks have taken up a central position in solution focused brief therapy. Tasks are framed in a way that presupposes change will occur, such as 'Notice what happens when you resist the urge to drink more than two pints', 'Notice what happens when you move one point further up your scale', 'Notice the signs of the miracle starting to happen'. This language matches that used when the therapist is interviewing in relation to goals and exceptions, for example, '*When* the problem is solved, *what* will be different between you both then?' '*When* are the times you are most able to resist the urge to go more than two pints?'

Observation tasks are especially valuable because they avoid the risk of the therapist devising a task that the client is, for whatever reason, unable to follow through on. This can result in a degree of tension entering the client–therapist relationship, as the client has 'failed' to do what was suggested by the 'expert', and the therapist has 'failed' to give the client the 'expert' advice. If the client reports in the next session that he or she hasn't noticed anything, then this is all that has happened: useful things might actually have happened, only the client didn't notice them – and so the search for exceptions goes on.

A well-known observation task developed by de Shazer became known as the First Session Formula Task (de Shazer, 1985):

Between now and the next time we meet, I would like you to observe, so that you can describe to me next time, what happens in your life that you want to continue to have happen.

This task was initially developed to enable clients who seemed particularly vague about their problems and their goals to start to define for themselves what was going well in their lives. Later this became the subject of a research study examining its usefulness when being applied to every case at the end of the first session. The study, conducted by de Shazer and his colleagues on a general population of clients (de Shazer, 1985.) showed that 89% of clients reported that something worthwhile had happened, and gave their reports in terms that were concrete and specific.

Two further tasks have been found to be of particular use with clients in the drug and alcohol field (Berg and Miller, 1992). As so many clients will report that the exceptions that have been identified are somehow beyond their control ('I don't know how I stopped drinking that day. I guess it was just the way I felt that day'), and as developing a sense of control is of such importance in enabling clients to repeat the behaviours that are good for them, then it is helpful to suggest observation tasks that will enable the clients to learn for themselves what it is they do on better days. One task is 'Between now and the next time we meet, I want you to notice what it is you are doing when you resist the urge to drink/to use'. The second task involves asking the client to predict at night whether they are likely to have a good or a bad day the next day, and to see if their prediction turns out right or wrong. They can then examine the difference between what they expected and what actually happened. The intention of this task is clear: clients are to assess the difference between their behaviours on the different days, so that behaviours that seem random and spontaneous to them can become deliberate and under their control.

Observation tasks 'work' therefore because they enable clients to become clearer about what is useful for them to repeat. It is even possible to ask clients to begin the observation process before the therapy has begun. The Milwaukee team (de Shazer *et al.*, 1986) found that two-thirds of a random sample of clients reported changes between the time the appointment was made and the time of the first session. It is therefore possible to treat the first telephone call as a first session and to ask the client to look out for changes before the first meeting. The changes then reported in the first meeting are referred to as pre-session change and are a valuable sign to client and therapist alike that change is able to take place – or at least that the client can cope better with his or her situation.

Ending therapy

In general, therapy ends when clients believe they have made sufficient progress towards their goals as stated in the earlier part of the therapy. A solution focused therapist treats each session as if it could be the last, and regards sessions after the first as essentially 'follow-ups' where exceptions are explored to highlight how the client is able to progress towards his or her goals. The client is asked if and when he or she would like to return.

If a client returns to report that things have actually been getting worse, the therapist will continue to search for exceptions and to explore what is helping the client to cope and survive. If things remain stuck the therapist will need to consider reclarifying the goals of the work.

At an earlier stage in the development of solution focused therapy it was not uncommon for therapists to ask some 'relapse prevention' questions, for example, asking what clients would do differently in future if they found themselves drinking again. This is much less common now. The general principle could be defined as the therapist having the job of helping clients initiate their own change-making behaviour . . . and then getting out of the way as quickly as possible.

Case illustration

A young woman called seeking an appointment for herself and her husband, who she stated had a drinking problem. At the first session it was apparent that her husband did not want to be there. His rather cryptic replies and negative body language conveyed that forcefully. His drinking history went back several years causing difficulties within the marriage, loss of jobs and friendships as well as contributing to financial hardship, particularly over the past year. In such a situation, where one member of a couple is reluctant to attend, the therapist explores their differing perspectives on the problem in such a way that a new perspective is allowed to come forth; one that might suggest a solution. Excerpts from this couple's initial session illustrate the kind of dialogue that often occurs when one, or both, members anticipate having to admit to having the problem.

> Therapist: So what would you think would be useful for us to talk about today?
> Husband: I just want to get out of here. I don't understand what all the fuss is about. I like to drink. She is against my drinking and blames it for everything.
> Wife: I'm fed up with it, I can't rely on him any longer for anything. It's as though he only cares about his friends and the pub.

From this brief excerpt, it is apparent that both the husband and wife have become quite adamant in their view that the problem lies with the other person. The interviewer then has to make it clear that it isn't his job to decide who or what is the problem.

Among other things, the couple speculate on each other's past history, on other examples of broken promises, as well their mutual concern that trust has gone out of the relationship. The need to air these bitter feelings, regarding the degree and nature of the problem, is quite common and reflects the tendency to blame the other person, believing that this is the solution to the problem. Switching back the therapist asked:

> Therapist (To the husband): What is it about drinking that you enjoy?
> Husband: I like to drink beer. I enjoy meeting my friends at the pub and there are times when I just like drinking socially with my wife.

The therapist then explored the same question from the wife's point of view, encouraging her to decide whether she wanted his drinking to stop altogether or whether she would be satisifed if they could just eliminate the problems.

> Wife: I'm not sure. I don't like complaining all the time, nagging. If I could be convinced that things could get better between us again I wouldn't care so much about his drinking.

Therapist: Uh huh.

Wife: If he came home after work more often and took an interest in things around the house, I could believe it could get better between us.

Therapist: What about your relationship at present; would you say it is OK, doesn't need to change?

Husband: I think there are plenty of things that are just fine.

Therapist: For example?

Husband: We have a laugh together. (Looks over at his wife)

Wife (With a hint of a smile): He's a practical joker. He can make me laugh when he wants to.

Therapist (To the wife): What would be a recent example of that happening?

Wife: About a month ago. We like to decorate; it's a bit of a hobby. When we moved in together we decorated his flat and later sold it. We did all right.

Husband: Yeah, and I wasn't drinking either.

The therapist was struck by how different the atmosphere had become, how both seemed less hostile and accusatory when talking about anything other than the problems they associated with the drinking. When pressed further, this line of enquiry produced several other examples of times that they agreed 'things were just fine'. They described, with good humour, times when they like to prepare meals for one another, as well as enjoying socialising in their home with friends.

At the end of the session the therapist complimented them on having provided clear examples of times when the problem wasn't interfering in their lives. He then asked them 'Between now and the next time we meet, look out for any additional examples of times when you are both getting along'. The couple responded quite enthusiastically to this suggestion and seemed quite prepared to carry it out.

When they returned for the next session the husband reported a considerable change in his drinking. Moreover, much to his surprise, his wife reported that there had been several significant changes, particularly in how they related to one another. While his drinking had not stopped, by this second session it was hardly focused on during the discussion. It may be that the 'knock-on effect' of the initial enquiry, regarding what the husband liked from his drinking, unlocked a series of examples of what the couple had valued in their relationship.

The therapist expressing an interest in the various aspects of the client's life that are working is an example of looking for exceptions: those times when the problem is not occurring or in some way less of a problem. In another case, a young cocaine user's response to the miracle question illustrates the potential to elicit information that can alter the client's perception from that of one immersed in the problem to one who sheds light on potential solutions.

Robert came to his initial interview with his sister. For most of the session they had taken turns describing the extent of the problem and how it was ruining Robert's life. Having listened attentively to the client's description of the problem Robert was asked the miracle question.

Therapist (asking slowly): Robert, imagine that tonight when you go home, while you're asleep, a miracle occurs and all the problems that brought you here tonight have been solved. As you are sleeping you won't know that this miracle has occurred until you've woken up. What is the very first thing that you would notice that tells you that a miracle had occurred?
    Robert (after a momentary pause): I wouldn't think about it. I'd take a shower, as I do every morning and I wouldn't think about cocaine in the shower.
    Therapist (writing this down): Ah! What else?
    Robert: I'd have something to eat. You know (laughing to himself) breakfast.
    Therapist (continuing to write): What else?
    Robert: I'd play with my boy. Get to work on time. Be more, what's the word, productive at work.
    Therapist: What would your sister notice about you that would tell her the miracle had occurred?
    Robert: Wouldn't fly off the handle; be less stroppy. Be interested in things.
    Therapist: What would your wife notice?
    Robert: Be more interested in doing things with her again, around the house; cleaning, you know.
    Therapist: Have any of these things already started to occur?
    Robert: Oh! Yeah. I took my son to work with me today. I had a good day at work; I wasn't feeling very good but I got along with everyone. I ate something this morning.

Robert's response is a good example of the importance of utilising the client's understanding of what will be happening when the problem is no longer there. By including the perspective of those close to him, Robert is able to contemplate the added beneficial effects to various relationships that need to occur. The fact that some of these changes are already happening helps emphasise his capacity to change, which may have gone unnoticed.
    Having summarised with Robert all of the points that he has mentioned would be different in his life without the problem, the therapist goes on to 'operationalise' the miracle by using a scaling question.

Therapist: I'd like to ask you a question with regard to all the things you've said would occur when the problems are solved. On a scale from zero to ten, with ten being all the things you mentioned the day after the miracle occurs, i.e. not thinking about cocaine, eating breakfast, playing with your son, getting to work on time, being more productive at work, less stroppy and more interested in doing things again; that is your ten. Zero is the point when things were at their worst. What number would you chose to represent where you are today?

Robert: A one.

Therapist: (writing down) So you see yourself as having already moved up to a one. OK.

Robert: Yeah, I've definitely got better. I've definitely moved from 0 to 1 in the last two weeks.

Earlier Robert had talked about details of the miracle picture that he was already seeing in his life. Through the scale question he is identifying the degree of change that he believes he has made. At the end of the session Robert was given positive feedback on all those aspects of his life that appeared to be helpful to him in moving forward. He was then asked to notice changes in his scale rating in the time up to the next session.

Conclusions

The underlying principle of solution focused brief therapy is the idea of the *exception*, that there are times when the problem is less or non-existent. This entails a view that clients have the resources and the competence to solve their problems, only their experience of failure has led them to discount or not even to notice the skills and influence they do have. Clinical activity consists in discovering and exploring exceptions.

The focus of the therapy is always towards the client's goals. All clients can be said to be customers for something, and it is essential for the therapist to co-operate with the client in identifying what those goals are. Only when they have been attained can the therapy be judged a success.

Success with such an approach leads to the view that in order for therapy to be successful it may not be necessary for the therapist (or the client) to know what the problem is. The movement of the therapy is in the direction of solution development, that does not entail exploring and understanding the history of the problem. It has therefore been found that there is little need to distinguish between the types of substance being used.

Our experience has been that individuals and families feel empowered when viewed as taking responsibility for change, and respond by facing up to issues of their drug use.

The research conducted on this approach indicates a high level of success. de Shazer reports (de Shazer, 1991) that a follow-up that ascertained the clients' own views regarding meeting their goals or making significant improvement found an 80.4% success rate within an average of 4.6 sessions. The results seem unaffected by such considerations as type of problem and length of its occurrence or whether it was the client's or someone else's idea that he or she has therapy. Similar results have been obtained in two very small pilot research studies conducted in this country (Iveson, 1991; Parslow, 1992). We do not, however, know of any study that has looked only at work with substance misusers.

References

Berg, I. K. and Miller, S. D. (1992) *Working with the Problem Drinker: A Solution-Focused Approach.* New York: Norton.

de Shazer, S. (1985) *Keys to Solution in Brief Therapy.* New York: Norton.

de Shazer, S. (1988) *Clues: Investigating Solutions in Brief Therapy.* New York: Norton.

de Shazer, S. (1991) *Putting Difference to Work.* New York: Norton.

de Shazer, S. (1994) *Solution Focused Brief Therapy.* Workshop Presentation, Brief Therapy Practice, 10/11 November, London.

de Shazer, S., Berg, I. K., Lipchik, E. *et al.* (1986) Brief therapy: Focused solution development. *Family Process,* **25**, 207–22.

George, E., Iveson, C. and Ratner, H. (1990) *Problem to Solution: Brief Therapy with Individuals and Families.* London: BT Press.

Iveson, D. (1991) *Outcome in Therapy.* MSc Dissertation. London: Birkbeck College.

Lethem, J. (1994) *Moved to Tears, Moved to Action: Solution Focused Brief Therapy with Women and Children.* London: BT Press.

Parslow, S. (1992) *On a Scale of 1 to 10: a different way of evaluating brief solution focused brief therapy.* MSc Dissertation, London: Birkbeck College.

Watzlawick, P., Weakland, J. and Fisch, R. (1974) *Change: Principles of Problem Formation and Problem Resolution.* New York: Norton.

9

Recent developments in cognitive and behavioural therapies

RUTH WILLIAMS

Introduction

The last 15 years have seen a rapid widening of therapeutic forces from the more specific anxiety disorders and other circumscribed problem areas that first occupied the behaviourists in the 1960s and 1970s to more complex problems such as depression, generalised anxiety, panic, hypochondriasis and so on. These developments owe much to the theoretical ideas of Beck (1976), which were originally applied to the treatment of depression (Rush *et al.*, 1977), and which have now been found to be generalisable to the treatment of wider if not all psychiatric disorders. Whilst effective for many patients (see Hollon *et al.*, 1992 for a review of outcome efficacy in depression and Chambless and Gillis, 1993 for a review of studies in anxiety), a significant proportion of patients do not respond to Cognitive-Behavioural Therapy (CBT), and much of the outcome variance is attributable only to unexplained and uncontrolled patient factors.

Along with the expansion of the range of problems treated there has been considerable recent interest focused on the 'difficult patient'. Developments have also occurred both in what Teasdale and Fennell (1982) called 'the delivery system', the way the therapeutic ideas are taught and are practiced by the patient, and in the theoretical ideas themselves and in the processes of therapy.

The present discussion will concentrate on developments in theory and therapeutic practice, presenting two approaches: the work of J. E. Young on personality disorder, and Linehan's very original therapeutic system, Dialectical Behaviour Therapy (DBT).

Schema-focused therapy (J. E. Young)

The background to Young's work (Young 1990; Young and Klosko, 1993) was his experience of working with patients with some different characteristics than those who had responded well to short-term CBT. He began encountering a group of patients whose problems were less severe or acute, who described less functional impairment, but who made little or no progress in standard CBT. These patients tended to be diagnosed as having long-term personality problems and were characterised by cognitive rigidity (a failure of beliefs to be influenced by contrary evidence), the use of avoidance strategies (cognitive, behavioural and affective) and the prominence of interpersonal problems, such as repetitive inappropriate choices of partners, overreactions to problems within the relationship, and so on.

Theory

To accommodate working within a cognitive framework with these patients, Young developed the concept of the Early Maladaptive Schema (EMS). The concept of a schema or Dysfunctional Assumption was originally used by Beck (1976) to explain the origins of specific negative automatic thoughts associated with emotional problems. A schema is a much-used term in various branches of psychology (Stein, 1992), although the meaning of the term may vary in different areas of application.

In Beck's usage, a schema is a cognitive structure, established in childhood, which allows the individual to select, interpret and respond to certain types of information automatically, without conscious attention. Such structures are essential to normal adult functioning but Beck hypothesised that some schemas may be laid down as a result of adverse early family or other environmental input, which are dysfunctional in that they are rigid, global, excessive and distort information processing. The final process of Beck's standard CBT is to identify and modify such dysfunctional assumptions using rational cognitive and behavioural techniques. Young has taken this concept and elaborated it, producing a taxonomy of the variety of schemas hypothesised to underlie personality problems, and describing the ways in which they function. The whole focus of the therapy, Schema-focused Cognitive Therapy, is upon identifying, dealing with and modifying these schemas.

Young defines EMSs in terms of 'important beliefs and feelings about oneself and the environment which the individual accepts without question' (Bricker and Young, 1993).

Rather than resulting from individual traumatic events, Young conceives of these structures as being formed as a consequence of the interaction of biological temperamental characteristics of the individual with repeated patterns of adverse experiences with family or others in the child's environment. For example, a child who is frequently criticised for failing to meet parental standards may form an 'incompetence' schema, a belief that he or she is not capable of coping alone with day-to-day demands. This belief may erupt when events occur that are relevant to it, for example, when the individual is faced with a task construed as difficult. Thoughts such as 'I can't. It's too much. I will fail' will be experienced together with a high level of anxiety. Since these beliefs are acquired early in life they are thought to form core aspects of the individual's identity and concept of the environment. They can be pre-verbal in form and are extremely resistant to change. They are dysfunctional in that they block the individual from meeting basic needs, for example, autonomy, connectedness, and self-expression. They also give rise to emotional problems and to addictions, psychosomatic disorders and other behaviours that hurt the individual, other people or both.

Whereas Young originally conceived of the EMS as differing from Beck's Dysfunctional Assumptions in being absolute and unconditional, developed at an earlier developmental period and tied to higher levels of affect when activated (Young, 1990), his more recent thinking is to subsume Dysfunctional Assumptions within the broader concept of the EMS (Young, 1994). Some of Young's taxonomy of beliefs, therefore, are more unconditional and some are more like Dysfunctional Assumptions or 'rules for living'. Clinical experience backed up by factor-analytic studies has resulted in a comprehensive list of 16 EMSs grouped into five categories corresponding to the hypothesised major developmental tasks that a child needs to negotiate, and which account for the range of personality problems encountered in the clinic. This taxonomy has undergone a variety of changes since 1990 and might be viewed as work in progress and awaiting replication. Young's theory is briefly summarised in Table 9.1.

Young attributes his choice of beliefs to no sources or influences. Inspection of the list confirms his recent account of EMSs as comprising a mix of both unconditional beliefs about the self and the world of others (Disconnection and Autonomy groupings) and problems with how to interact with the environment (Impaired Limits, Other-Directedness and Overvigilance/Inhibition). The former groupings are similar in content to Beck's concepts of autonomy and sociotropy as personality vari-

Table 9.1 *Young's early maladaptive schemas (1994)*

---

1. *Disconnection and rejection* – expectation that one's needs will not be met by others in a reliable fashion
   Abandonment/instability – others are perceived as unreliable
   Mistrust/abuse – others will abuse
   Emotional deprivation – need for emotional support will not be met
   Defectiveness/shame – self is bad, unloveable, defective
   Social isolation/alienation – self is isolated, different

2. *Impaired autonomy and performance* – expectation that one will not be able to survive/perform independently
   Dependence/incompetence – self is unable to handle responsibilities of everyday living without help
   Vulnerability to random events – random catastrophe may occur at any time
   Enmeshment/undeveloped self – self is excessively involved with another at the expense of individuation
   Failure – self has failed, will inevitably fail in areas of competence

3. *Impaired limits* – deficiency in internal limits, responsibility to others or long-term goal orientation
   Entitlement/domination – self should be able to do or have anything
   Insufficient self-control/self-discipline – difficulty in exerting self-control or frustration tolerance to achieve goals

4. *Other-directedness* – excessive focus on others at expense of personal needs
   Subjugation – surrendering control under coercion from others
   Self-sacrifice – excessive giving up own needs for the sake of others
   Approval-seeking – self must have approval from others

5. *Over-vigilance and inhibition* – excessive focus on self-control to avoid mistakes or to meet internal standards, at expense of personal needs
   Vulnerability to controllable events/negativity – exaggerated expectation that things will go wrong
   Overcontrol – excessive inhibition of spontaneous behaviour
   Unrelenting standards – self must meet internal standards
   Punitiveness – self is intolerant of failure in others

---

ables (Beck *et al.*, 1983). These concepts occur in many theoretical ideas about self-concept and self-esteem (e.g. Coopersmith, 1967; Epstein, 1973). Impaired Limits, Other-Directedness and Overvigilance groupings seem more similar to the Dysfunctional Assumptions of Beck and colleagues: for instance, the unrealistic should/must/need beliefs about how an individual is to live to avoid global negative evaluation (Kovacs and Beck, 1978). Factor analysis of the Dysfunctional Attitude Scale (Weissman and Beck, 1978), the most commonly used measure of this construct, has yielded a number of factors relating to, for example, perfectionism, the needs for approval or to please others, self-punitiveness and control over emotions, which are similar in content to some of Young's EMSs.

Empirical support

Studies of thinking about the self in children add some validity to the theory of EMSs. Harter (1990) has studied developmental changes in concepts of self in children, from the concrete behavioural descriptions of young children, to more abstract descriptions of psychosocial variables, to the multiple facets and differentiation in mature adults. Studying the development of concepts of competency, Harter observed that younger children typically evaluate themselves in global and all-or-nothing terms. This judgment is normally positive but global and absolute, but global negative judgments have been found in children in therapy for learning problems (Harter, 1985). Thus, there is some evidence for early global and undifferentiated beliefs about the self. Harter also points out that different developmental stages of abstraction and differentiation may occur with respect to different life domains, and that earlier developmental forms may remain in the repertoire rather than drop out. Thus, mature ways of thinking may exist with respect to some concepts, and within concept to some domains of application.

Schema processes

Young describes three processes by which the EMS functions. **Schema maintenance** is the process by which the schema resists disconfirmatory information by means of cognitive distortions, for instance by minimising information that is inconsistent with the belief. For example, a student dismisses evidence that he or she is intelligent by explaining away accomplishments as due to chance factors. **Schema avoidance** arises because the emotions experienced when a schema is active are very intense and unpleasant. The individual therefore develops a range of strategies to stop this happening that include cognitive avoidance (attempts to avoid thinking about the content of the schema), affective avoidance (blocking the emotional response to schema material), and behavioural avoidance (avoiding situations or activities that might trigger the schema). **Schema compensation** is the process by which the individual overcompensates for the presence of the schema by acting in an extreme way to contradict its assumptions. For example, a person throws him or herself into excessively demanding work to prove that he or she is competent. All these processes have the effect of maintaining the individual's belief in the schema and creating strong resistance in therapy when questions are raised about the schema's validity.

Therapy

The processes of Schema-focused Cognitive Therapy differ in some important ways from Beck's approach. There is much more emphasis upon the therapeutic relationship, upon examining how interpersonal problems are elicited in therapy, and using the relationship to promote change. Young describes therapy as involving a limited re-parenting experience for some patients. There is also much more emphasis upon events in the past, and especially childhood relationships, from a rational point of view to reframe childhood experiences, and from an experiential point of view to activate and change schema derived from childhood. Young says that rather than using exclusively rational approaches for the control of excessive emotions as in standard cognitive therapy, there is a greater need with these patients to elicit and work with emotion itself. He allows an important place within therapy for the release of stored up emotions. As one might expect, the duration of the therapy is longer, possibly a year or 18 months.

Interpersonal aspects

Because of schema maintenance processes, Young considers simple 'collaboration' with the patient as not sufficiently powerful. Schema avoidance, for example, may result in patients being unaware of the problems they have in some areas. Young encapsulates the essential nature of the therapeutic relationship in schema-focused therapy as 'empathic confrontation'. He uses the EMS conceptualisation of the patient's problems as a tool in the understanding and acceptance of the patient but takes up a strong position upon the necessity to confront the processes of schema maintenance so as to accomplish change. He uses the metaphor of the 'devil inside you' to distance the patient from identification with the schema assertions, and exhorts the patient to engage in a battle to defeat the schema.

Assessment and initial techniques

The process of schema-focused therapy begins with an assessment phase during which the therapist conceptualises the patient's problems, present and life-long, in terms of EMSs and schema processes. This formulation is then shared with the patient. Young uses convergent multiple assessment methods in arriving at the formulation, including interview techniques focusing upon problems, and on childhood and life experiences with a view to EMS issues. He also uses the Lazarus and Lazarus (1991) Multimodal Life-History Inventory, and has constructed a 205 item Schema Questionnaire to assess self-reported belief in the 15 EMSs. The additional source of information is the patient's in-session behaviour with the therapist with a view to schema issues.

An interesting part of the assessment phase is the use of open-ended and focused imagery to elicit schemas and to test out the formulation. Links between childhood and current feelings are made by asking the patient to switch from a childhood image to a present situation 'that feels the same'. The assessment phase is interspersed with education about the concepts of therapy, using written material as well as in-session discussion.

Young cautions about using the more direct and focused methods with fragile patients (specifically severe obsessive-compulsive, borderline, abuse victims and post-traumatic stress disordered patients), and recommends always leaving adequate time at the end of the imagery sessions to de-brief, talk about the schemas, to ground the patient in the present and prepare for emotions arising outside of sessions.

Change techniques

Young categorises the methods of change in schema-focused therapy as cognitive, experiential or emotive, interpersonal and behavioural. Cognitive techniques, similar to those used in standard cognitive therapy, are used to test the evidential basis of EMSs in the present and in the past. Therapist and patient can role-play imaginary dialogues between a schema and the patient's 'healthy side', with the aim of developing the patient's ability to use arguments to defeat the schema's reasoning. Useful lines of argument can be written down on flashcards for the patient to refer to at times when the schema is active out of session.

Young uses more experiential or emotive techniques to uncover suppressed emotions resulting from childhood memories that form the basis of the EMS. For example, a woman who had an emotional deprivation schema was encouraged to express the feelings of pain and anger that she had experienced in the past, in an imaginary dialogue with a parent. The result of this experience may be that the patient can further reconstrue the meaning of these experiences, understand why they happened, and put them into the past.

Interpersonal techniques are used to highlight the way in which schemas perpetuate themselves in behaviour with current partners who reinforce the role of the schema. This process can be explored in relation to in-session behaviour with the therapist, or partners may themselves be involved in the process of discovering more functional ways to think and behave.

Finally, behavioural techniques may be used to overcome self-defeating behavioural patterns that reinforce schemas through acting in ways that allow the patient to obtain core needs without hurt to others. Examples of such behavioural techniques are assertiveness training, choosing partners who do not mesh with EMSs, and communications skills training. Young describes this behavioural change phase of therapy as the most lengthy.

Comment

Young has developed the theory and methods for dealing with basic beliefs in cognitive therapy and these ideas have received a great deal of professional interest in recent years. His ideas owe some provenance to the work of Millon (1981) and Guidano and Liotti (1983). The therapy process also bears some similarity to Cognitive Analytic Therapy described by Ryle (1989). The use of imagery to pin-point dysfunctional beliefs provides a method that may increase the speed and the accuracy of CBT. But we have yet to see these ideas subjected to the crucial test of empiricism, both with respect to the theoretical basis or to the outcome of therapy. If it were indeed possible significantly to modify entrenched beliefs associated with maladaptive personality characteristics within the space of one year, then Young's ideas would be a major therapeutic breakthrough. Clearly there are problems in measuring relatively 'soft' symptoms and changes in interpersonal behaviour but the field definitely needs at least some uncontrolled case studies to have continuing credibility.

Young's ideas also have some disadvantages. It is problematic to have two systems of cognitive therapy, one for emotional disorders and one for personality problems. Many patients presenting for therapy probably have both types of problem and it is notoriously difficult to establish the nature of enduring personal problems in the presence of an Axis 1 disorder. It is not completely clear that the 'schema' therapy is, in fact, to be regarded as a new therapy rather than an elaboration and extension of methods of working with basic beliefs in cognitive behavioural framework. Many therapists have incorporated Young's methods comfortably within an overall CBT framework (Gilbert, 1992).

There is a suggestion in Young's thinking and in the field generally that the self-controlling techniques of standard cognitive therapy may feed into the maladaptive beliefs of some patients, and this idea requires serious consideration. Several outcome studies have shown a bi-modal response to cognitive therapy and we urgently need better selection criteria in view of the scarcity of this therapeutic resource. One testable hypothesis is that high scores on Young's Over Vigilance and Control Schemas could predict poor outcome on standard cognitive behavioural treatment, for which the more emotive techniques of Young's approach could be indicated. However, by endorsing too readily the schema approach, we may be in danger of throwing out the baby with the bath-water and too casually dismissing the value of rationality in dealing with emotional distress without putting it to the test.

Another disadvantage of Young's method is the loss of the collaborative relationship. This has been the principal guardian against therapist bias in a therapy that goes beyond behaviour into the realm of the subjective. It is also a highly attractive feature of cognitive therapy to those who mistrust the dogmatism of some therapeutic approaches. Young's method carried with it an increased danger of getting it wrong, putting ideas into people's heads when they are in a vulnerable state, and of alienating them. It is easy to overvalue ideas formed from in-session behaviour. Young admits that drop outs occur, mainly in the assessment stages of therapy, and it is easy to see how this might happen with the strength of some of the metaphors used and the confrontative stance. It is also easy to see how a patient's disagreement with the therapist's formulation could be taken as 'resistance' and only further evidence of the formulation's validity.

Dialectical Behaviour Therapy (DBT) (Linehan, 1993)

Linehan's unique work (Linehan, 1993) with chronically parasuicidal women reaching criteria for Borderline Personality Disorder (BPD) is not widely known outside the USA, but is notable for the outcome results recently published with this hard-to-help and deeply distressed group.

Theory

Linehan bases her therapy upon a dialectical world view: dialectical in assuming the interrelatedness of the parts of the world, in assuming that the world is not static but comprised of opposing forces out of the

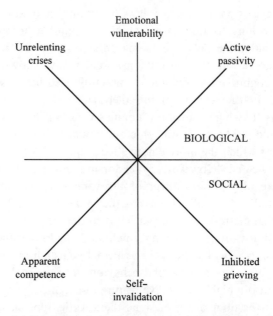

Figure 9.1 Borderline behaviour patterns (after Linehan, 1993).

syntheses of which new opposing forces emerge. A major axiom is that the truth is paradoxical and contains within itself contradictions. Linehan applies the notion of dialectics to borderline psychopathology by hypothesising that the patient is stuck with extreme polarities of opposing feelings, thought, and behaviours, and is unable to make the move to their syntheses. Such a theory is compatible with the schema approach of Young, with the addition that in the borderline patient different schemas may be conflictual, and lacking internal consistency and coherence.

Linehan characterises borderline patients' behaviour as showing three dimensions represented by their dialectical poles (Figure 9.1). Dividing each pole by its mid-point, one half is hypothesised to arise more from biological influences and the other from social factors. The patient is seen as caught between the opposing poles of emotional vulnerability versus self-invalidation, active passivity versus apparent competence, and unrelenting crises versus inhibited grieving.

Theoretical Axes

Emotional vulnerability is a major component of the biological stratum of Borderline Personality Disorder in Linehan's system. This consists of high sensitivity to emotional stimuli, high emotional intensity and slow habituation. Linehan (1993) says that the borderline patient is the 'psychological equivalent of the third-degree burn patient. They simply have, so to speak, no emotional skin'. She also points out how difficult it is for the therapist to keep this vulnerability in mind, when it is often hidden. **Self-invalidation** is the patient's adoption of the stance of his or her social environment. He or she attempts to inhibit emotional reactions, oversimplify life's problems, distrust his or her own perceptions and react with self-hate in the face of the failure of these strategies to be effective. Linehan points out that this polarity within the patient poses a difficult dilemma for the therapist because both sympathy and understanding *and* attempts to induce change, can be seen by the patient as invalidating, and may constitute the basis for angry attacks on the therapist, or drop-out, or suicide attempts. Linehan's solution is to employ both strategies and flexibly to adjust the approach between acceptance and change with moment-to-moment agility, a dialectical balancing act.

Active passivity is approaching a problem in a passive and helpless style, whereas **apparent competency** is acting as if coping skills are intact, the latter often to the fore when the patient is in the reassuring presence of the therapist. The discrepancy acts to perpetuate the invalidation the patient receives from the environment, and prevents the therapist from offering needed skills training and more gradual shaping of achievements. Equally, it is easy for the therapist to underestimate coping skills, particularly when suicide is on the agenda, and fall into the trap of helping the patient out and reinforcing the patient's helplessness. Again, therapy can be seen as a dialectical balancing act, flexibly alternating between support and gradual shaping of change.

The dialectic between **unrelenting crises** and **inhibited grieving** represents both the continually stressful life of the borderline patient, his or her over-reaction to every stressor, the environmentally led failure to learn and use coping skills in the face of invalidation and the use of avoidant strategies. Linehand points out the difficulty the therapist has in attending sensitively to each life-event dislocation and also carrying through a programme of skills teaching. Linehan solves this problem by utilising a skills session, group or individual, in parallel with individual therapy, where a programme of basic cognitive behavioural skills can be followed through.

The role of the individual therapist is thereby somewhat reduced to helping the patient to implement and practice skills rather than teaching them as well.

Therapy

Linehan divides treatment methods into four groups: dialectical strategies, core strategies, stylistic strategies and case management strategies.
These are represented in Table 9.2. The core strategies, problem solving
and validation incorporate the principal content materials of the therapy
whereas the dialectical strategies describe the pervasive methods whereby
the balance is achieved between acceptance and change. Stylistic strategies describe the interpersonal communication methods used in therapy.
Case management strategies describe the way in which the therapist inter-
acts with the patient's social network. These will be discussed in more
detail.

Core strategies

Validation
Defining 'validation' as the main acceptance strategy, Linehan (1993)
states (p. 223):

The therapist communicates to the patient that her responses make sense and are
understandable within the context of her current life context or situation. The
therapist actively accepts the patient and communicates this acceptance to the
patient. The therapist takes the patient's responses seriously and does not discount or trivialize them. Validation strategies require the therapist to search for,
recognise and reflect to the patient the validity inherent in her responses to events.

Specific methods include providing opportunities for emotional expression, helping the patient to observe and label in detail components of
emotional responses, reading the patient's emotions, recognising the

Table 9.2 *Dialectical behaviour therapy treatment methods (from Linehan, 1993)*

1. Dialectical strategies	⎰ Within therapeutic relationship
	⎱ Modelling dialectical responses
2. Core strategies	⎰ Problem solving
	⎱ Validation
3. Stylistic strategies	⎰ Reciprocal
	⎱ 'Irreverent' communication
4. Case management strategies	

'kernel of truth' in the patient's responses, offering developmental explanations for emotional responses, countering the patient's 'should' statements about his or her behaviour or emotions, helping the patient to identify the construction he or she is placing upon events, acknowledging the validity of differing values, encouraging the patient, focusing on his or her capabilities, taking up the position of an ally and communicating that the therapist is in support and stays near at hand.

Problem solving

Problem solving is highlighted as the general method of change. Linehan interprets suicidal behaviours as attempts to solve problems. The method therefore encourages the identification of the problems for which suicide is the problematic answer. Problem-solving strategies use methods familiar to cognitive-behavioural therapies: behavioural definition of problems, detailed functional analysis of problems, generation of hypotheses about variables that may influence or control behaviours to be tested out, education about the processes of change, identification of goals, generation of solutions and evaluation of solutions. Solution implementation will, for instance, include training, exposure strategies, cognitive modification, contingency modification, and case management depending upon the outcome of functional analysis. Linehan stresses that what is different in treating patients with borderline personality disordered patients is the necessity to repeat these stages many times. She also gives some added attention to the processes she refers to as 'orienting to therapy' and 'commitment' strategies. These methods orient the patient and therapist to their respective roles in therapy and generate commitment. Initially, the commitment may be just to work towards reducing suicidal behaviour. Linehan emphasises that commitment to this goal is the basic requirement for staying in therapy. Later in therapy, commitment is elicited with regard to specific treatment procedures such as skills learning and implementation of identified solutions to problems.

Cognitive-behavioural analysis will provide answers that guide the therapist in selecting change procedures. Inappropriate or inconsistent reinforcement from the environment suggests that contingency management is indicated. Linehan has discussed in some detail the issue of observing therapist's limits under this category. She suggests that therapists should be alert to detect behaviours of their patients that cross their own personal limits, and make these explicit to the patient promptly.

These behaviours are treated as the second most important problems to address in therapy (second only to suicide or self-harm). She observes that this is necessary because if not dealt with the therapist will terminate therapy, 'burn out' or otherwise harm the patient. She observes that personal limits will vary, and vary within individuals at different times. Suicidal threats are clearly particularly stressful. She points out that the therapist should give the patient good warning of the likely results of breaking their limits when the consequences are extreme (for instance, involuntary hospitalisation), and should provide the patient with a way to avoid such outcomes.

Other skills that may be chosen for implementation are emotion regulation, interpersonal effectiveness, distress tolerance and 'mindfulness' skills. The latter Linehan incorporates from Zen teaching as a method of dealing with the deficient sense of identity and emptiness often experienced by the borderline patient. The patient is taught quasi-meditational techniques that involve observing, describing and participating with a view to developing a sense of awareness, and an ability to step back from an event. Other mindfulness skills include the ability to verbalise about events and responses, and to participate in an event spontaneously and with awareness but without self-consciousness.

Stylistic strategies

The stylistic strategies used in DBT refer to the form of communications between therapist and patient rather than the content. There are two communication styles: the **reciprocal communication** is characterised by warmth, responsiveness, genuineness and self-disclosure. Linehan points out that many patients with BPD are very antagonistic to the unreciprocal power balance in some psychotherapies, and often alternate between needy subservience and domineering and dismissive behaviour in relationships. DBT attempts to establish a more equal relationship between therapist and patient, and personal self-disclosure forms a component of this strategy. The therapist will, for example, discuss his or her own attempts to deal with problems, and will seek to normalise the experience of problems and of coping and failure. Linehan, however, is careful to place this therapist behaviour in the context of there being a staff consultation team available to monitor and help the therapist in managing disclosure.

The second communication style is less easy to define and although this is apparently an important aspect of DBT, Linehan (1993) devotes little space to discussing it. She calls it '**irreverent communication**', and describes its function as providing the patient with vital psychological distance, and the ability to stand back and observe:

Keeping the individual just off balance enough to shake up her typically rigid, narrow-bounded approach to life, to herself and to problem-solving. The idea is to high-light both poles of the dialectic without denying either.

Case-management strategies

Case-management strategies concern how the therapist relates to people in the environment who have dealings with the patient. They include, for instance, consulting the patient about dealing with others, environmental interventions directly with others to help them understand and deal with the patient, and therapist supervision. The former two components are vital to consider when maladaptive behaviour is being reinforced by the social environment, and when adaptive behaviour needs to be noted and reinforced if change is to occur. Linehan's therapy manual contains, for example, detailed and systematic procedures for recommending ancillary treatments, avoiding or arranging hospital admissions, and for dealing with suicidal threats.

Linehan considers the supervision of therapists an integral part of the therapy programme. Interestingly, she draws again on the dialectical principal to counter the intense disagreements between team members that tend to arise in the treatment of these patients. She encourages a policy where all individuals look for the syntheses that integrate opposing views. The supervision team also operates to encourage and problem-solve with individual therapists.

Empirical support

Linehan and her colleagues have evaluated the effectiveness of their therapeutic programme in a controlled trial with a 12-month follow-up (Linehan *et al.*, 1991, 1993). Forty-four women between the ages of 18 and 45 years, who met criteria for BPD with parasuicidal behaviour, were randomly allocated to 12 months of DBT (3.5 hours therapy per week with 24 hour availability of telephone contact), or 'treatment as usual' in the community. Status was assessed at pre-treatment and 4, 8, and 12 months after entering the trial, on measures of frequency and medical severity of parasuicidal behaviours, psychiatric in-patient care, current suicidal ideation, depression, hopelessness and current reasons for living. Ratings were carried out by assessors blind to treatment allocation.

Frequency of parasuicidal acts was significantly lower in the DBT group at all follow-up points. DBT also maintained significantly more patients in therapy over the treatment period. DBT patients had significantly fewer days of psychiatric in-patient care. No significant differences were found on questionnaire measures of depression, suicidal ideation, hopelessness and reasons for living.

The results of the naturalistic follow-up study (Linehan *et al.*, 1993) broadly showed that differences were maintained over the second year, whether or not patients stayed in therapy. This study was carried out on the suicidal behaviour of 39 subjects. Both frequency of parasuicidal acts and hospitalisation were lower in the DBT group in the interval 12–18 months after cessation of treatment. Psychiatric admission rate was also significantly less in the 18–24 month interval after the end of the experimental period. At both time points the experimental group scored higher on measures of employment adjustment and global adjustment. At 18 months, DBT subjects also reported less anger and better overall social adjustment. At 24 months, DBT subjects were rated more highly on overall social adjustment. The authors concluded that they had demonstrated a significant treatment effect in a study with relatively low statistical power, but did not claim a 'cure'.

Comment

Linehan's work represents the only treatment approach of this kind that has been subject to controlled evaluation to yield a specific, significant treatment effect with this patient group, and therefore deserves scrutiny. In her manual, Linehan demonstrates both systematic attention to detail and an overarching system within which the detail is placed. With respect to the detail, Linehan has, in the writer's view, captured the basics of what individual cognitive behavioural therapy is about. She has been able to spell out precisely what with most patients it is natural to do, but which is all too easily disrupted by the Borderline patients' interpersonal behaviour. There is no doubt in this reviewer's mind that this work is the result of long and hard experience with these patients. Every eventuality is catered for. The amount of therapeutic time involved in the therapy system can be argued as justified by the difficulties in standard therapy that these patients present. The whole system of individual therapy, weekly skills training, 24-hour availability of therapist and consultation team, gives a realistic notion of what it requires to break into these patients' schemata. It would, however, be a brave therapist who attempted a replication. And it has to be accepted that although there are changes in behaviour over a year's DBT, subjective experiences are only slightly affected, or at least measurement only picks up a slight effect.

Although the change interventions are mainly within the behavioural sphere and reinforcement issues have an important place, it is interesting to consider the unique cognitive component in Linehan's treatment and to compare with Young. Linehan disagrees with the insistence on challenging distortions in thinking in standard cognitive behavioural treatment, whereas Young takes a strong confrontative position on 'fighting' the schemas and engaging the patient's healthy self in the battle. Possibly Linehan is more concerned than Young to keep her patients in therapy (and alive). Linehan may also be less sanguine about the existence of a healthy side because of her view of the Borderline patient as stuck between opposites, rather than stuck with a stable negative view of the self that is activated on occasion. Her intention is to help the patient to integrate across apparently contradictory parts of experience. Perhaps a more explicit cognitive educational component to the therapy could facilitate this integration.

Another interesting comparison is the difference in the use of developmental material between the two approaches. Borderline patients often report a history of abuse, and Linehan's theoretical position about the role of invalidation in the environmental contribution to BPD might lead one to suppose that the understanding of the past might play an important part in therapy. Linehan is clear that patients must learn the skills of emotional regulation before such issues can be dealt with in therapy, and such work would therefore not feature during the first year of therapy. Young is less concerned about the patient managing intense emotions outside of sessions and would probably concur that his very direct and emotionally arousing methods would be unwise early in therapy with a patient prone to impulsive self-harm.

Finally, it is interesting to compare the relationship styles advocated by the two therapeutic systems. Young is educative, prescriptive and confrontational and claims considerable expert knowledge in the extent to which he will intervene in the patient's life. Linehan is perhaps more sophisticated and subtle, aiming to flatten the power gradient between patient and therapist and present the therapist as an equal and as a supporter (a 'cheer leader') although also as a facilitator of change.

Ways ahead

This selective review of contrasting recent advances in theory and technique in CBT for personality problems reveals the extent to which cognitive-behavioural therapists are being more adventurous in the exploitation of the therapeutic relationship as a vehicle for change in therapy. They also reveal the more recent commitment to using emotion-eliciting techniques in therapy as opposed to techniques to reduce and contain emotional arousal. The former obviously have a greater risk attached and are not advised for dealing with those who have few coping skills. These developments have led some to question whether personal therapy should be a requirement for therapists working within this style (Annual Conference of the British Association of Behavioural and Cognitive Therapies, 1994.) These methods do certainly make considerable personal demands upon therapists in the way they deal with interpersonal issues arising in-session. One cannot assume that all CBT therapists have the relevant skills.

Clearly the overlap between the theories and methods of these CBT advances and traditional psychodynamic therapies are striking, and provide some support for the emergent integrative movement. The testing out of these approaches, which have much face validity to many contemporary clinicians, is awaited with interest.

References

Beck, A. T. (1976). *Cognitive Therapy and the Emotional Disorders*. New York: International Universities Press.

Beck, A. T., Epstein, N. and Harrison, R. (1983). Cognitions, attitudes and personality dimensions in depression. *British Journal of Cognitive Psychotherapy*, **1**, 1–16.

Bricker, D. C. and Young, J. E. (1993). *A Client's Guide to Schema-Focused Cognitive Therapy*. ATID publications.

Chambless, D. L. and Gillis, M. M. (1993). Cognitive therapy of anxiety disorders. *Journal of Consulting and Clinical Psychology*, **61**, 248–60.

Coopersmith, S. (1967). *The Antecedents of Self-esteem*. San Francisco: W. H. Freeman.

Epstein, S. (1973). The self concept revisited or a theory of a theory. *American psychologist*, **28**, 405–16.

Gilbert, P. (1992). *Counselling for Depression*. London: Sage.

Guidano, V. F. and Liotti, G. (1983). *Cognitive Processes and Emotional Disorders*. New York: Guilford Press.

Harter, S. (1985). Competence as a dimension of self evaluation: towards a comprehensive model of self-worth. In: Leahy, R. (ed.) *The Development of the Self*, pp. 55–122. New York: Academic Press.

Harter, S. (1990). Developmental differences in the nature of self-representation: implications for the understanding, assessment and treatment of maladaptive behaviour. *Cognitive Therapy and Research*, **14**, 113–42.

Hollon, S. D., Shelton, R. C. and Davis, D. D. (1992). Cognitive therapy for depression: conceptual issues and clinical efficacy. *Journal of Consulting and Clinical Psychology*, **61**, 270–5.

Kovacs, M. and Beck, A. T. (1978). Maladaptive cognitive structures in depression. *American Journal of Psychiatry*, **135**, 525–33.

Lazarus, A. and Lazarus, C. N. (1991). *Multimodal Life History Inventory*. Illinois: Research Press.

Linehan, M. (1993). *Cognitive-Behavioural Treatment of Borderline Personality Disorder*. New York: Guilford Press.

Linehan, M., Armstrong, H. E., Suarez, A., Allmon, D. and Heard, H. L. (1991). Cognitive-behavioural treatment of chronic para-suicidal, borderline patients. *Archives of General Psychiatry*, **48**, 1060–4.

Linehan, M., Heard, H. L. and Armstrong, H. E. (1993). Naturalistic follow-up of a behavioural treatment for chronically parasuicidal borderline patients. *Archives of General Psychiatry*, **50**, 971–4.

Millon, T. (1981). *Disorders of Personality*. New York: Wiley.

Rush, A. J., Beck, A. T. and Kovacs, M. (1977). Comparative efficacy of cognitive therapy and pharmacotherapy in the treatment of depressed out-patients. *Cognitive Therapy and Research*, **1**, 17–37.

Ryle, A. (1989) *Cognitive-Analytic Therapy: Active Participation in Change (A New Integration in Brief Psychotherapy)*. London and New York: Wiley.

Stein, D. J. (1992). Schemas in the cognitive and clinical sciences: an integrative construct. *Journal of Psychotherapy Integration*, **2**, 45–63.

Teasdale, J. D. and Fennell, M. J. V. (1982). Cognitive therapy with chronic drug-refractory, depressed out-patients: a note of caution. *Cognitive Therapy and Research*, **6**, 455–60.

Weissman, A. and Beck, A. T. (1978). *Development and Validation of the Dysfunctional Attitude Scale*. Paper presented at the Annual Convention of the Association for Advancement of Behaviour Therapy, Chicago.

Young, J. E. (1990). *Cognitive Therapy for Personality Disorders: A Schema-focused Approach*. Florida: Professional Resource Press.

Young, J. E. (1994). *Schema-focused Cognitive Therapy*. Workshop for the British Association of Behavioural and Cognitive Therapies, London, UK.

Young, J. E. and Klosko, J. S. (1993). *Reinventing Your Life*. New York: Dutton Books.

10

Cognitive and behavioural treatments for substance misuse

MICHAEL GOSSOP

Assessment and goal setting

Assessment is an important first stage of treatment. It should not be relegated merely to the role of an impersonal procedure to be completed prior to treatment. Just as the drinker or drug-taker is actively involved in his or her own addictive behaviour, so they must be actively involved in their own recovery. It is the responsibility of the therapist to use assessment as an important opportunity to encourage that involvement. Indeed, it may be more appropriate to regard this first stage of treatment as reaching a mutual agreement about goals rather than simply setting goals.

Psychology has always had a primary interest in behaviour, and among the general themes of psychological treatments for addiction problems two prominent issues have been the focus upon the psychosocial context in which drug-taking occurs, and the targeting of interventions at addictive *behaviour*. Psychology has also shown a particular interest in the *antecedents* of the overlearned habits that are the addictions, including the situational and environmental circumstances in which the behaviour occurs, the beliefs and expectations of the user, and his or her prior learning experiences with the drug itself. In addition, psychology has an equal interest in the *consequences* of these behaviours, and specifically in the reinforcing effects that may lead to increased use and the negative consequences that may serve to inhibit the behaviour.

Traditional types of assessment procedures for behaviour modification programmes as described by Kanfer and Phillips (1970) have been found to be directly applicable to the treatment of addictive behaviour. Information is needed about target behaviours, the reinforcement parameters maintaining them, opportunities in the environment for maintaining other more desirable responses, and the individuals' ability to observe and reinforce themselves.

For all types of drug problems that require treatment, the intervention offered should be tailored to the needs and circumstances of the individual. This apparently simply and uncontentious statement turns out to have complex and far-reaching implications for policy and services if it is seriously applied in clinical practice (Gossop, 1987). There is not, nor can there be expected to be, any single best treatment for these problems. Both aetiology and outcome are influenced by a broad range of different factors that will differ in important respects from person to person. It is essential that a thorough assessment should identify, *for each individual case*, the nature of the problem and appropriate and achievable goals for treatment. Also, the treatment process should identify as early as possible those particular factors that are likely to assist or hamper the achievement of the treatment goal(s).

Examples of types of treatment goals might include the following:

1. Reduction of psychological, social or other problems not directly related to the drug problem.
2. Reduction of psychological, social or other problems that are related to the drug problem.
3. Reduction of risky behaviour associated with the use of drugs.
4. Attainment of controlled or non-dependent drug use.
5. Attainment of abstinence from problem drug.
6. Attainment of abstinence from all drugs.

These six examples are not mutually exclusive. Treatment goals may include the attainment of abstinence as well as the improvement of psychosocial functioning in areas unrelated to drug-taking. It is, however, useful to distinguish between those treatments that are *directly* focused upon addictive behaviour as a treatment goal and those that have an indirect, theoretical or hypothesised relationship to addictive behaviour as a goal. It has been part of psychology's contribution to draw attention to the importance of targeting addictive behaviour directly. For many years the majority of treatments for addictive behaviours were misdirected against hypothetical intrapsychic faults or underlying personality disorders. These 'ghosts in the machine' were presumed to be both causes of the addiction and obstacles to recovery. As a result, the choice of treatment goal and the focus of treatment became that of personality restructuring. The addictive behaviour was neglected on the grounds that it was no more than the mere symptomatic expression of the underlying problem that would correct itself once the more 'profound' disorder was successfully treated. One consequence of this sort of approach was that treatment tended not only to be unfocused but also endless.

The possibilities of applying treatment goals other than abstinence – and in particular that of helping people with alcohol problems to regain control over their drinking – has proved to be a controversial issue. Much of this controversy has been generated by groups who have denied on *a priori* grounds that alcoholics can regain any control over their drinking. However, the issue can also be regarded as a problem of the practical feasibility of treatment matching. It is generally accepted that not all alcoholics will be able to regain control over their drinking, and there is some suggestion that those who are able to do so may be a comparatively small minority. Pattison (1976) suggests that the proportion of alcoholics who develop normal drinking patterns either after treatment or after changes in their social circumstances may be between 10 and 15%. As a result, many clinicians continue to support abstinence as a general treatment goal on the grounds that the attempt to predict which individuals will be successful in regaining control over their drinking remains little more than guesswork. 'So long as no one knows what it takes to reactivate [alcoholism] in any individual who is addicted . . . the prudent alcoholic in remission should not put himself on trial' (Keller, 1972). Some studies have suggested that moderate drinking is more likely to be an appropriate goal for moderately dependent, than for heavily dependent alcoholics (Orford *et al.*, 1976), and that the patient's attitude to controlled drinking, their age, employment and pre-treatment patterns of drinking may be important selective factors (Heather and Robertson, 1981), but beyond these rather general observations there is little empirical evidence or sound theory to which the clinician can turn for guidance.

Concern about HIV infection among drug injectors has provided a powerful impetus to the acceptance of non-abstinence treatment goals in the treatment of illicit drug problems. A variety of 'harm reduction' treatments are now used with drug-takers and the application of goals other than abstinence to the treatment of heroin and opiate addiction has often been linked to drug substitution treatments such as methadone maintenance. The provision of maintenance drugs has been shown to be effective in many cases, though the strength of the evidence supporting methadone maintenance has sometimes been overstated (Gossop, 1978*a*). There is, however, a sufficient core of evidence to support the suggestion that some addicts will show improvement in other areas of their life if given a controlled supply of maintenance drug. Some of the most difficult long-term opiate addicts attending a London drug clinic showed improvements in social functioning after being prescribed an increased dose of opiates (Gossop *et al.*, 1982*b*), and in a comprehensive investigation of methadone maintenance in the United States, Ball and Ross (1991), provided compelling evidence of the benefits of this type of treatment.

Treatment approaches

Stages of change

Prochaska and DiClemente (1986) described several stages of change that can be applied to an understanding of addictive behaviours. These stages are **Precontemplation, Contemplation, Decision, Action** and **Maintenance.** This model and its later developments are discussed at length in Chapter 12.

Precontemplation is a stage in which people do not intend to change their behaviour. Individuals in this stage are not aware or are not sufficiently aware that they have problems, though others (family, friends, doctors) may be acutely aware of this. When precontemplators approach treatment services it is usually because they are under pressure from others. Contemplation is the stage in which the individual shows an awareness of his or her problem and begins to think about making changes but without a serious commitment to take action. People may be stuck in the contemplation stage for long periods.

After making a decision to change, the action stage involves actual attempts to modify behaviour, experiences and/or environment in order to overcome addiction problems. People, including professionals, often equate change with action and consequently overlook the important work that prepares individuals for action. During the maintenance stage the individual works to prevent relapse and consolidate gains. However, it is unlikely that the actual processes of change will involve any orderly progression through the different stages. It is also often clear that some people with addictive behaviour problems may become stuck in one or other of the stages.

This sort of model can be useful in drawing attention to the different factors that may be appropriate to the different processes and stages of change and it can serve as an important guide to therapists. For example, patients in the precontemplation stage should be helped to recognise and develop an awareness of their problems rather than being guided directly towards behavioural change. Patients in the contemplation stage are most open to consciousness-raising interventions (such as self-monitoring procedures or educational methods) and may be resistant to the interventions of a directive action-oriented therapist. During the action stage patients are likely to require practical help with behaviour change procedures as well as encouragement and support. Preparation is required both for action and for maintenance. It is interesting that therapists as well as patients can become stuck in a favoured stage of change.

The question of motivation

The term *motivation* has a murky history in relation to the treatment of addictive behaviours. Einstein and Garitano (1972) pointed to the circularity in the way that this term has been so often misused p. 235:

The general approach is that if the drug abuser patient gets better – translated that means he gives up his drugs of choice – he was a good and motivated patient and was able to profit from our professional expertise and skill. We cured him. If the patient continues his drug use, this is manifest evidence that he was not motivated, and a poor treatment risk who could not profit from our skill.

This circularity has been a major factor in leading to a dissatisfaction with the concept of motivation. However, it may not be necessary completely to reject the term. It can be rescued from circularity and it can be shown to relate to treatment response. When motivation is operationally defined (for example, in terms of the strength of the addict's desire for treatment), this is an important determinant of how long addicts subsequently remain in treatment (Gossop, 1978b). However, motivation should not be seen as an unchanging or as an entirely 'internal' factor and the extent to which it changes in response to external social and environmental factors requires further clarification.

In recent years, the term has re-emerged in relation to a form of treatment known as 'motivational interviewing' (Miller, 1983). This has been found to be a useful tool in many stages of treatment but it has been particularly useful in helping people with substance abuse problems who are still ambivalent or even resistant to change (such as precontemplators). Since motivation and motivational treatments for the addictive behaviours are addressed elsewhere in this volume they will not be discussed any further in this chapter (the reader may turn to Chapter 11).

Relapse: the problem and its prevention

One of the most influential models of treatment in recent years has been Relapse Prevention. Perhaps the best-known version of this has been described by Alan Marlatt and his colleagues (e.g. Marlatt and Gordon, 1985). Relapse Prevention may be seen as a self-management programme designed to enhance the maintenance stage of the process of change. The primary goal of Relapse Prevention is to teach individuals who are trying to change their drug-taking behaviour how to identify, anticipate, and cope wth the pressures and problems that may lead towards a relapse. The foundations of Relapse Prevention work are the notions of high risk situations and the coping strategies available to the individual.

The process of relapse has been studied among alcoholics (Litman, 1980) and among heroin addicts who had recently completed in-patient treatment (Gossop *et al.*, 1989). Many of these former addicts were found to use opiates again in the period immediately after leaving treatment. Eighty-one per cent used opiates at least once during the six-month period, and in most cases, the lapse occurred very soon after discharge. The time immediately after leaving treatment is a critical period during which recovering addicts are at extremely high risk. Almost two-thirds of those who lapsed indicated that cognitive factors, usually some explicit decision or plan to return to opiate use, were implicated in their initial lapse. More than half indicated that some negative mood state (sadness, boredom, tension or anxiety) preceded their lapse. These associated factors occasionally occurred as single relapse precipitants, but more often they occurred as clusters – several simultaneous relapse factors, or as sequences – one or more factors leading on to others (Bradley *et al.*, 1989).

One contribution of these studies of relapse has been to draw greater attention to the clinical significance of relapse as a process in its own right and to the factors outside treatment that influence outcome. There has also been undue emphasis on the problem of cessation of drug use, when what is required is more emphasis on the difficulties encountered in maintenance of the change once cessation has occurred. Craving and urges might be triggered by environmental or by internal cognitive cues, and an important first task for the client is to develop an awareness of the way in which these triggers may contribute towards the development of a high-risk situation. Clients may be encouraged to keep regular diaries detailing use of drugs and the extent to which they have encountered possible precipitants of relapse and a summary of their response. The therapist will assist them to conduct a behavioural analysis of these situations to teach the clients how to conduct such a behavioural analysis themselves. Structured problem-solving techniques are employed along-side rehearsal or role play. The client is warned of the dangers of the way in which covert planning may lead to relapse, and of the way in which decisions may 'by chance' lead the client to be confronted by high-risk situations. The client must learn to spot early warning signals for those potential relapse situations.

Special interventions should be applied as indicated by assessment and feedback from the client. Where addiction problems are related to under-lying anxiety disorders, treatment will involve the application of treat-ment techniques that are appropriate to anxiety management. Where deconditioning of craving is required, the clinician will be guided by the same principles and apply the same procedures that would be appro-priate, for instance, to systematic desensitisation of phobic states. Where the acquisition of new behavioural coping skills is required the therapist will attempt to achieve this in the same way as with any other type of patient.

Brief interventions

One of the most interesting developments in recent years has involved the application of brief interventions with people who have drinking or drug problems. The types of brief intervention have varied but have often involved either the provision of reading materials or simple advice and information. A series of studies conducted by Miller looked at the uses of self-help manuals for heavy drinkers and concluded that such methods could be effective (e.g. Miller *et al.*, 1981). Since the early studies of Miller, others have developed and evaluated such methods. In the UK, Heather *et al.* (1986) evaluated the impact of a similar manual (*So You Want to Cut Down Your Drinking?*) and found that drinkers who had received the manual had made significant reductions in their drinking and reported fewer alcohol problems than a control group. Such methods often emphasise the issues of self-monitoring of drinking behaviour with functional analysis, and self-control with self-reinforcement and alternatives training (Miller and Hester, 1980).

One of the larger and more recent studies of brief interventions was carried out by the WHO as a cross-national multicentre clinical trial (Babor and Grant, 1991). Of the 1490 eligible patients who were recruited at eight centres, 75% were subsequently followed up. This trial investigated the impact of simple advice and brief counselling upon alcohol consumption, and it was conducted with heavy (but not severely dependent) drinkers. Its rationale was to detect and intervene with people with harmful alcohol consumption before health and social consequences became pronounced. The results of this trial were described as very promising and showed that various brief interventions, ranging from five minutes of simple advice to 20 minutes of advice plus counselling, can produce a significant reduction in alcohol consumption. Even the briefest intervention (simple advice from a family doctor) was found to be an effective way of helping people to cut down their drinking.

Although these studies of brief interventions have been with alcoholics, there is no reason why these methods and procedures should not be adapted for use with drug addicts, and the application of brief intervention methods to drug problems presents an interesting challenge for the future.

Conditioning treatments

Attempts have been made to apply conditioning principles to the behavioural treatment of dependence disorders and cue exposure methods have attracted much attention in recent years. The origins of such methods date back to the earliest studies of Pavlov in which it was shown that animals can acquire responses to stimuli that had previously been associated with drug effects. Abraham Wikler recognised that the self-administration of heroin (or other opiates) by drug-takers is associated with many environmental variables, such as the sight and smell of the drug itself, the rituals surrounding drug-taking, specific locations, etc. These acquire the properties of discriminative stimuli in operant conditioning. The same variables tend also to be paired with the abstinence effects and become classically conditioned to these environmental stimuli (Wikler, 1980). Drug-seeking and drug-taking behaviours are powerfully reinforced thousands of times during the course of a person's drug-using career.

Examination of the role of classical conditioning in the experience of drug effects and subsequent dependence has produced apparently conflicting findings. Conditioned euphoria may occur in the presence of drug-related cues (O'Brien and Childress, 1991). However, there is also convincing evidence that the abstinence syndrome can be conditioned as a response to specific environmental stimuli in both animals and man

(Wikler, 1980). Subsequent study has demonstrated the role of both unconditioned and conditioned drug effects as reinforcers (Stewart *et al.*, 1984).

The application of cue exposure methods has an important role in the treatment of phobic and obsessive-compulsive behaviour where they are variously referred to as flooding, exposure, participant modelling and response prevention (Hodgson, 1982). Such forms of treatment rely upon the idea that a strong urge to carry out a compulsion will go away if the urge is resisted.

In a clinical setting, the patient is exposed to cues (identified during assessment, and possibly including drug-related cues such as the sight of injecting equipment, social cues such as meeting other drug users, or internal cues such as anxiety or boredom) which would usually have triggered an episode of drinking or drug-taking. During this exposure session, the patient may be supervised, may be in a protected environment in which there is no access to drink or drugs or may (in the case of alcohol) have previously taken an aversive drug such as disulfiram. The aim is to break down the stimulus–response relationship that has developed to the drug and to various conditioned stimuli, by exposing the patient to the stimuli in sessions when these are not associated with reinforcement through drug-taking. This approach may be used to achieve abstinence, but it has also been used as part of programmes aimed at controlled drinking (Heather and Robertson, 1981).

In work with methadone-maintained opiate addicts, Childress *et al.* (1984, 1988) demonstrated habituation of subjective craving, and the clinical status of addicts who received cue exposure treatments was encouraging at follow-up. Other work done with people dependent upon cocaine (Childress *et al.*, 1988) showed significant responses to cocaine-related cues after 28 days cue exposure treatment. However, the clinical uses of cue exposure have not been fully established. A recent clinical trial of cue exposure treatments for opiate addicts at the Maudsley Hospital in London provided the most stringent clinical trial of cue exposure yet conducted with this client group. Cue exposure was found to produce no significant improvement in rates of abstinence nor in time to relapse when compared to standard treatment methods (Dawe *et al.*, 1993). All addicts showed a significant reduction in cue reactivity and this occurred independently of cue exposure treatment. For the moment, such treatments must be regarded as of unproven efficacy with regard to the treatment of opiate addiction. In the Maudsley trial, the authors concluded that these results 'do not invalidate the theoretical basis of cue exposure treatment, but we have major reservations about its practical value'.

Psychological and physical aspects: a caveat

Drug addicts and alcoholics may suffer from various forms of physiological impairment that interfere with or prevent effective psychological treatment. The cortical atrophy found among heavy drinkers is associated with difficulties in concentration, and in its later stages produces a state indistinguishable from senility. Drug users with HIV infection may develop an AIDS encephalopathy or AIDS dementia complex with problems ranging from mild cognitive deficits to full-blown dementia. Clearly in such advanced cases there are huge obstacles to conducting any therapeutic programme that requires complex and integrated psychological skills. However, it is not fully known to what extent the less severe states of neurological impairment may interfere with the patient's ability to understand, remember and carry out the requirements of therapy (Glass, 1991).

The fact that a condition is primarily physiological in nature does not, though, in itself preclude psychological intervention. The most immediate medical feature of treatment is often the detoxification of the user. Many drugs, notably heroin and other opiates, produce physical dependence such that the addict suffers from withdrawal symptoms when he or she stops taking the drug. This is true of the barbiturates and the benzodiazepines, and alcohol too has a serious withdrawal syndrome. Many addicts are anxious about the prospect of withdrawal and anxiety may serve to increase levels of discomfort during withdrawal (Phillips *et al.*, 1986).

In this context, the provision of factual information about the duration and severity of withdrawal, and about the type of withdrawal symptoms that will occur, has been found to significantly reduce the distress reported by heroin addicts during detoxification and to increase detoxification completion rates (Green and Gossop, 1988). This simple procedure may be seen as one instance of how a brief intervention can usefully be applied to the treatment of drug addiction.

Treatment in perspective

The traditional answer to the question 'How good are treatments for addictive behaviours?' has tended to be pessimistic, for instance that 'a small proportion of alcoholics achieve abstinence within six and 12

months of receiving treatment, whatever the nature, intensity and duration of the treatment concerned' (Clare, 1977). An earlier review of treatments for drug addiction reached a similar conclusion: 'There is no
relationship between time spent in treatment and the outcome of treatment. There is no relationship between the type of treatment and the
outcome of treatment. Whoever the agent of therapy is, whether he be
the aggressive social worker, the Rogerian counsellor, the pastoral counsellor, the psychoanalytically oriented psychotherapist, the clinician who
uses methadone maintenance, or the ex-addict giving mutual aid, the end
result is not significantly different. The great majority of addicts simply
resume drug use' (Einstein, 1966).

Such pessimism is no longer warranted. There is now an impressive
weight of evidence from recent research that shows that even people with
severe dependence upon drink and drugs can recover from their addictions (Biernacki, 1986; Gossop *et al.*, 1989; Strang *et al.*, 1990). In many
respects, it is atypical for addicts to remain addicted throughout their
lives. The majority will give up at some point.

The negative expectations about the role of treatment in producing
change are due, at least in part, to a misreading of the evidence about
lapses after treatment (Gossop, 1988), and from confusion about the role
that treatment might have in assisting the process of recovery.
Treatments for drug and alcohol problems often provide only a relatively
small input to the world of the drug-taker or drinker. Also, it is important
for the clinician to acknowledge that intentional change, such as occurs in
therapy, is only one type of change (Prochaska and DiClemente, 1986).
Developmental and environmental changes can also be responsible for
people changing their patterns of drug or alcohol consumption. As in the
aetiology or development of drug problems, the psychology of the individual and the social setting in which the individual lives exert powerful
influences upon outcome. For the therapist, in the treatment setting, it
may be tempting to believe that treatment factors are more powerful than
they really are.

However, it can be equally misleading to underrate the potential input
of factors outside the treatment context. Hubbard *et al.* (1989) note that
'The role of treatment is to change behaviours and psychological states
and to direct clients to community resources during and after treatment',
and that 'Programmes have no direct control on behaviour after clients
leave treatment. Rather, treatment should influence post-treatment behaviour indirectly through changes in psychological states and behaviour
during treatment' (p. 35). In this sort of model, treatments directed at the

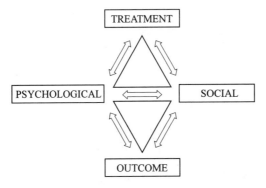

Figure 10.1 Effects of treatment, psychological and social factors upon outcome.

maintenance of change after treatment should be seen as operating indirectly upon the target behaviour through their ability to change the factors that influence outcome (see Figure 10.1).

Edwards (1989) also offered a warning about the limitations of treatment and suggested that excessive enthusiasm about treatment effectiveness can be misguided; this enthusiasm can be 'constrained to the point of tunnel vision if it assumes that treatment influences are so paramount that all that has to be asked is "Does treatment work?" with every other influence . . . discounted . . . Treatment is more accurately conceived as being at best a timely nudge or whisper in a long life course'.

Several important treatment outcome studies have been published recently. Moos *et al.* (1990) looked at the context, process and outcome of treatments for alcoholism. They concluded that treatment led to substantial improvements in drinking behaviour. The study also looks carefully at how much of the outcome variance can be attributed to pre-treatment personal factors, intensity and quality of treatment, and the family and wider social context. The evidence about treatment impact is more encouraging than that reported in many studies though individual and social factors also played an important role in determining outcome.

In the field of drug problems, the Treatment Outcome Prospective Study (TOPS) involved more than 11 000 people who entered treatment for drug problems at 41 treatment programmes in the United States (Hubbard *et al.*, 1989). Samples were interviewed at three months, one year, two years, and three to five years after leaving treatment. The study showed substantial decreases in the abuse of opiates and other drugs after treatment. Reductions in drug-taking continued up to three to five year follow-up. Interestingly, in relation to the increased awareness of applying cost/benefit analysis to treatment, the TOPS study demonstrated the 'substantial crime-related and other costs . . . of drug abusers prior to treatment and the substantial reductions in these costs both during and following participation in treatment'.

References

Babor, T. and Grant, M. (1991) *Project on Identification and Management of Alcohol-Related Problems: Report on Phase II. A Randomized Clinical Trial of Brief Interventions in Primary Health Care*. Geneva: World Health Organisation.

Ball, J. and Ross, A. (1991) *The Effectiveness of Methadone Maintenance Treatment*. Springer: New York.

Biernacki, P. (1986) *Pathways from Heroin Addiction*. Philadelphia: Temple University Press.

Bradley, B., Phillips, G., Green, L. and Gossop, M. (1989) Circumstances surrounding the initial lapse to opiate use after detoxification. *British Journal of Psychiatry*, **154**, 354–9.

Childress, A. R., McLellan, A., Ehrman, R. and O'Brien, C. (1988) Classically conditioned responses in opioid and cocaine dependence: a role in relapse? In: Ray, B. (ed.) *Learning Factors in Substance Abuse*. NIDA Monographs, **84**, 25–43. Washington.

Childress, A. R., McLellan, A. and O'Brien, C. (1984) Measurement and extinction of conditioned withdrawal-like responses in opiate dependent patients. In: Harris, L. (ed.) *Problems of Drug Dependence*. NIDA Monographs, **49**, 212–9, Washington.

Clare, A. W. (1977) How good is treatment. In: Edwards, G. and Grant, M. (eds.) *Alcoholism, New Knowledge and New Responses*, pp. 279–89. London: Croon Helm.

Dawe, S., Powell, J., Richards, D. *et al.* (1993) Does post-withdrawal cue exposure improve outcome in opiate addiction? A controlled trial. *Addiction*, **88**, 1233–45.

Edwards, G. (1989). As the years go rolling by. Drinking problems in the time dimension. *British Journal of Psychiatry*, **154**, 18–26.

Einstein, S. (1966) The narcotics dilemma: who is listening to what? *International Journal of the Addictions*, **1**, 1–16.

Einstein, S. and Garitano, W. (1972) Treating the drug abuser: problems, factors and alterations. *International Journal of the Addictions*, **7**, 321–31.

Glass, I. (1991) Alcoholic brain damage: what does it mean to patients? *British Journal of Addiction*, **86**, 819–21.

Gossop, M. R. (1978*a*) A review of the evidence for the effectiveness of methadone maintenance as a treatment for narcotic addiction. *Lancet*, **i**, 812–5.

Gossop, M. R. (1978*b*) Drug dependence: a study of the relationship between motivational, cognitive, social and historical factors, and treatment variables. *Journal of Nervous and Mental Disease*, **166**, 44–50.

Gossop, M. R. (1987) What is the most effective way to treat opiate addiction? *British Journal of Hospital Medicine*, **38**, 161.

Gossop, M. (1988) Addiction and after. *British Journal of Psychiatry*, **152**, 307–9.

Gossop, M. R. and Connell, P. H. (1983) Drug dependence: who gets treated? *International Journal of the Addictions*, **18**, 99–109.

Gossop, M. R., Eiser, J. R. and Ward, E. (1982*a*) The addicts' perceptions of their own drug taking: implications for the treatment of drug dependence. *Addictive Behaviours*, **7**, 189–94.

Gossop, M., Green, L., Phillips, G. and Bradley, B. (1989) Lapse, relapse and survival among opiate addicts after treatment. *British Journal of Psychiatry*, **154**, 348–53.

Gossop, M., Strang, J. and Connell, P. (1982*b*) The response of outpatient opiate addicts to the provision of a temporary increase in their prescribed drugs. *British Journal of Psychiatry*, **141**, 338–43.

Green, L. and Gossop, M. (1988) Effects of information on the opiate withdrawal syndrome. *British Journal of Addiction*, **83**, 305–8.

Heather, N. and Robertson, I. (1981) *Controlled Drinking*. London: Methuen.

Heather, N., Whitton, B. and Robertson, I. (1986) Evaluation of a self-help manual for media recruited problem drinkers. *British Journal of Clinical Psychology*, **25**, 19–34.

Hodgson, R. J. (1982) Behavioral psychotherapy for compulsions and addictions. In: Eiser, J. R. (ed.) *Social Psychology and Behavioral Medicine*, pp. 375–91. London, New York: Wiley.

Hubbard, R., Marsden, M., Rachal, V. *et al.* (1989) *Drug Abuse Treatment: A National Study of Effectiveness*. Chapel Hill and London: University of North Carolina Press.

Kanfer, F. and Phillips, J. (1970) *Learning Foundations of Behaviour Therapy*. New York: Wiley.

Keller, M. (1972) On the loss of control phenomenon in alcoholism. *British Journal of Addiction*, **67**, 153.

Litman, G. (1980) Relapse in alcoholism. In: Edwards, G. and Grant, M. (eds.) *Alcoholism Treatment in Transition*, pp. 294–304. London: Croon Helm.

Marlatt, G. A. and Gordon, J. R. (1985) *Relapse Prevention*. New York: Guilford.

Miller, W. R. (1983) Motivational interviewing with problem drinkers. *Behavioural Psychotherapy*, **11**, 147–72.

Miller, W. R., Griboskov, C. and Mortell, R. (1981) The effectiveness of a self-control manual for problem drinkers with and without therapist contact. *International Journal of the Addictions*, **16**, 829–39.

Miller, W. R. and Hester, R. (1980) Treating the problem drinker: modern approaches. In: Miller, W. R. (ed.) *The Addictive Behaviors*, pp. 11–141. Oxford: Pergamon.

Moos, R., Finney, J. and Cronkite, R. (1990) *Alcoholism Treatment: Context, Process and Outcome*. New York: Oxford University Press.

O'Brien, C. and Childress, A. R. (1991) Behaviour therapy of drug dependence. In: Glass, I. (ed.) *Addiction Behaviour*, pp. 230–5. London: Routledge.

Orford, J., Oppenheimer, E. and Edwards, G. (1976) Abstinence or control: the outcome for excessive drinkers two years after consultation. *Behaviour Research and Therapy*, **14**, 409–18.

Pattison, E. M. (1976) Non-abstinent drinking goals in the treatment of alcoholism. *Archives of General Psychiatry*, **33**, 923–30.

Phillips, G., Gossop, M. and Bradley, B. (1986) The influence of psychological factors on the opiate withdrawal syndrome. *British Journal of Psychiatry*, **149**, 235–8.

Prochaska, J. and DiClemente, C. (1986) Toward a comprehensive model of change. In: Miller, W. and Heather, N. (eds.) *Treating Addictive Behaviors*, pp. 3–27. New York: Plenum.

Stewart, J., de Wit, H. and Eikelboom, R. (1984) Role of unconditioned and conditioned drug effects in the self-administration of opiates and stimulants. *Psychological Review*, **91**, 251–68.

Strang, J., Gossop, M. and Stimson, G. (1990) Courses of drug use: the concepts of career and natural history. In: Ghodse, H. and Maxwell, D. (eds.) *Substance Abuse and Dependence*, pp. 80–97. Basingstoke: Macmillan.

Wikler, A. (1980) *Opioid Dependence*. New York: Plenum.

11

Motivational issues in the treatment of addictive behaviour

ROBIN DAVIDSON

Introduction

The outcome of any therapy depends not only on the use of appropriate treatment strategies but also on how persistently and conscientiously the patient carries them through. It is the tenacity of the individual in pursuit of his or her chosen goal that is a crucial factor in long-term success. Heather (1992) put it succinctly when he commented that 'addictive disorders are essentially motivational problems'. The therapist is more than just a dispenser of appropriate treatments or a donator of advice. The therapist must act as a catalyst to help unravel the motivational forces that contribute to the persistence of old self-defeating behaviours or, alternatively, the intiation and maintenance of new more adaptive ones.

The word motivation comes from the Latin root meaning 'to move' and is an attempt to understand what moves us or why we do what we do (Wade and Tarvis, 1992). It is an inferred set of processes, which cause a person to move towards a particular goal. Miller (1985) gives us a practical definition of motivation as the 'probability that a person will enter into, continue and adhere to a specific change process'.

There has been considerable debate among psychologists over the years on how best to account for the complexity of human motives. The early focus on instincts gave way to drive theory (Hull, 1943), which dominated our thinking in the mid-twentieth century. However, this approach did not full take account of the interaction between socially learned motives and biological needs. Festinger's (1957) work began to bridge this gap with his ideas on cognitive balance and dissonance leading to an understanding of the human motives to organise and deal with experiences in terms of a more general belief system. Later McClelland (1961) noted that forces like the need for competence, predictability, achievement, or power, can fuel our goal-directed journey. The historical development of general motivational theories within psychology is, however, beyond the scope of this chapter.

The following section examines the background of some cognitive interventions which have become popular in the addictions literature. It is argued that these are best understood in motivational terms. The discussion then focuses on ambivalence, which is particularly important in the light of contemporary motivational interventions developed for the treatment of addiction. Finally, given Miller's (1985) definition noted above, no discussion of motivation would be complete without reference to attrition in relation to treatment programmes.

Social cognition and motivation

Social cognition is the study of how information about oneself and others is registered and processed. The phrase 'social learning theory' was first coined by Dollard and Miller (1950) but contemporary authors generally use it when referring to the work of Bandura (1977) and Rotter (1975) on expectations. This is only part of the array of ideas that constitute social cognition. This body of work demonstrates that people behave because they believe certain outcomes will accrue, have belief systems that help consolidate and explain, make decisions, plan goals and plot strategies. Learned social motives are a key influence in determining the intensity and persistence with which a person performs a particular behaviour.

The sometimes oblique relationship between cognitive theory and therapy has been dealt with more fully elsewhere (Davidson, 1994) and is the subject of Chapter 9 in this book. Dobson (1988) identified over 20 different types of cognitive behaviour therapy, some of which are not necessarily grounded on experimental research in cognitive and social psychology. Furthermore, specific cognitive therapies seem to be applied in particular groups of presenting problems. In his attempt to integrate cognitive behaviour treatments within an information processing framework, Brewin (1989) suggested that there are three types of fundamental cognitive changes. First, therapists can rectify misconceptions in a person's accessible knowledge base. This process underlies treatments for disorders like panic, sexual problems, insomnia, stuttering and the like. The second type of cognitive change involves modifying access to nonconscious situational memories and this is central, for example, to Beck's (1976) approach of modifying dysfunctional assumptions associated with depression or generalised anxiety. The third type of cognitive change involves conscious appraisal of options and encouraging persistence in their use. It is this last group of cognitive approaches to behavioural tenacity and change that has dominated the addiction treatment literature. Brewin (1989) has described this third set of interventions as primarily enhancing *motivation* for coping behaviours and it includes strategies like re-attribution, expectancy training and problem solving.

The explanation or attribution theories can be traced to the ideas of social psychologists like Heider (1958) and Lewin (1947). Attribution theorists assume that the individual deliberately attempts to explain events in order to maximise future control and particular types of explanation are said to enhance behavioural persistence in the face of adverse circumstances. As an example of this work, Weiner's (1985) model of motivation and emotion falls squarely within an attribution/explanation framework. He argues that the way an individual accounts for a successful outcome produces optimism about future successes, and results in greater behavioural tenacity and intensity. The model posits that attributional hypotheses differ on three main dimensions, the most important of which in the present context is stability/instability. Stable attributions are those in which the cause is seen as a result of relatively permanent and unchanging characteristics of the individual. If we attribute a successful outcome to relatively enduring factors this then raises expectations of future success and accordingly greater behavioural persistence. If, however, successful outcomes are seen in terms of unstable factors, this produces a tendency to 'give up trying'. More recently, Davies (1992) has specifically applied attributional principles to drug use, and he argues that if this behaviour is seen as a result of personal and enduring characteristics, it mitigates against future change for the better.

Theories that emphasise expectancy and value can trace their roots back to early cognitive psychologists like Tolman (1948), and these have been particularly influential in the addiction treatment literature (Marlatt and Gordon, 1985; Annis and Davis, 1989). Bandura's (1985) work would suggest that the most successful therapies are those that encourage efficacy beliefs. The point here is that the self-efficacy theory is not concerned about why people become depressed, addicted, or fearful, but rather why they do not cope equally successfully with their problems. It is not the acquisition but the maintenance of problem behaviours that is central to Bandura's work, and so self-efficacy theory too is motivational in emphasis. Outcome expectations have been less mentioned in the alcohol treatment literature (Leigh, 1989), although in motivational terms they are as important, if not more so, than beliefs about efficacy. There is increasing evidence of an association between the balance of positive and negative outcome expectancies and future drinking behaviour. A particular type of outcome expectation is the placebo effect, without mention of which any discussion on motivation would be incomplete. Occasionally when 'successful' psychological interventions are compared with credible control procedures, their superiority can disappear completely (Lick and Bootzin, 1975). Russell *et al.* (1976) found that for smokers a technically incorrect behavioural programme was just as effective as one that was correctly implemented. There is much evidence that outcome expectations are part of any psychological therapy, and it is not useful to consider placebo as synonymous with 'inert' or 'non-specific'.

Other common interventions adapted for addictions from social cognition theories include those that promote self-regulation, for instance self-instructional training and problem solving. These too are also primarily focused on enhancing motivation for coping behaviours.

It could be said, therefore, that most post-behavioural therapies developed in addictions involve some combination of explanation, expectancy, contingency estimation or self-regulation strategies, and so arguably can be understood in motivational terms. Because of the operational complexity and ubiquity of motivational ideas in our treatment literature, the next section narrows the discussion more specifically to the area of motivational conflict. This is when satisfaction of one motive leads to an inability to pursue another. It is this idea of motivational conflict or ambivalence that is central to our understanding of change in addiction.

Ambivalence

Within addiction counselling, Davies (1981) noted that the motivational problems can be best understood in terms of patient ambivalence. Others like Miller and Rollnick (1991) and Bennett (1993), in their discussion of motivational interviewing, would see working with ambivalence as working at the very core of the problem.

Understanding of ambivalence has a long history in both the psychoanalytic and cognitive behaviour literature. Bleuler first used the word ambivalence in 1911 when he defined three types. Voluntary ambivalence is a conscious conflict about doing one thing versus something else. Intellectual ambivalence is a simultaneous interpretation of experience in positive and negative ways. Emotional ambivalence specifically refers to the feelings of love and hate directed at the same object. Freud (1913) built on this idea of emotional ambivalence as a precursor of defences like splitting and reaction formation (Holder, 1975).

Behavioural theorists have developed ideas broadly in line with Bleuler's conception of voluntary ambivalence when describing approach-avoidance conflicts. Sincoff (1990) summarised this work in her definition of ambivalence as 'overlapping approach avoidance tendencies, manifested behaviourally, cognitively or affectively and directed towards a given person or experience'. When defined in this way, ambivalence can result in personal distress, and more importantly perhaps the inability to make important life decisions. Janis and Mann (1977) illustrated how rational decisions should be made and decisional conflict is the 'simultaneous opposing tendencies within an individual to accept or reject a given course of action'. They argued that resolve comes about when losses arising from behaviour exceed the gains, thus prompting an individual to seek out new solutions.

Decisional conflict can be seen as an instance of ambivalence. In order to begin dealing with ambivalence, Abelson and Levi (1985) pointed out that the reluctant decision-maker must first determine when the information is relevant, second he must gather the information, and third he must integrate it in such a way that a decision can be reached. Abelson and Levi (1985) suggested that various obstacles to these steps can include information overload, lack of emphasis on the essential information, over-emphasis on non-essential information, and poor integration of information from various sources. This may lead to a sense of hopelessness, vacillation, and hesitation, thus promoting short-term solutions at the expense of long-term goals. What they term 'vigilant information processing' can reduce uncertainty, promote good decision-making, and minimise post-decisional regret. Vigilant information processing involves identification and examination of all viable alternatives, re-examining these in the light of new information and then specifying in advance the optimum ways of making a decision.

The obvious criticism of these cognitive models of conflict and ambivalence was articulated by Sloan (1986), who pointed out that they lean heavily on logic by ignoring self-reflection and subjective meaning of the decisions. Psychoanalysts would argue that ambivalence is symptomatic of more deeply rooted conflicts, which should be dealt with before indecision can be resolved. Sincoff (1990) made a plea that even cognitive therapists should explore with their ambivalent patients the dangers and threats to self that conflict resolution may involve.

Although there is no theoretical connection between ambivalence and 'purpose of life', one could be forgiven for speculating about an inverse relationship between the two. Frankl (1969) suggested that all people have a 'will to meaning', which can be defined as a basic striving to find and fulfil meaning and purpose, the frustration of which can lead, among other things, to substance abuse. Later, Newcomb and Harlow (1986) demonstrated that one correlate of successful alcohol treatment is a reported increase in a sense of purpose and a reduction of the 'existential vacuum'. Although the 'Purpose of Life' attitudinal scale seems something of an oxymoron, Waisberg and Porter (1994) have recently demonstrated that a higher score on this scale is associated with certain positive changes among former alcoholic in-patients. Perhaps this reported 'general change in outlook' among these individuals is part of a less ambivalent style of conflict resolution.

Ambivalence – state or trait

Our understanding of ambivalence as a trait, or alternatively as a situational variable, will impact on our understanding of change in addictive behaviour. Current treatment approaches emphasise the situational nature of ambivalence. Implicit in the decision balance model is that if the pros outweigh the cons, the individual is more likely to approach a decision than avoid it. Writers on motivational interviewing constantly emphasise that the presence of motivational conflict is not a personality problem and those who deny the need for change are not inherently lacking in motivation (Miller and Rollnick, 1991). Rather, denial is seen as a by-product of traditional confrontative interventions. By attempting actively to persuade a patient that a problem exists the therapist can be met with a 'yes but' response. Denial is therefore part of the therapist/patient dialogue rather than a stable characteristic.

Miller (1985) provided a comprehensive critique of the motivational literature. To view poor motivation, he argued, as a constitutional deficit is to foster expectancy of poor prognosis in patient and client. Leake and King (1977) elegantly demonstrated this point in a study which informed alcohol counsellors that a randomly selected group of patients had the potential for doing very well in therapy. These patients were subsequently rated by counsellors as more motivated, more committed to the treatment programme, and indeed this group actually did better than a control group after a year. This study also, quite graphically, demonstrates the power of therapist motivation in influencing change. Furthermore, if a client believes that poor motivation is a trait, then failure to change will be an internal stable attribution possibly reducing the chances of future success.

However, when we focus more specifically on motivational conflict or ambivalence, the picture is less clear. In the general psychology literature the state versus trait question is far from resolved. It can be argued that for some people ambivalence is not invariably situationally determined, but is a dispositional feature that admittedly becomes more strongly apparent in some specific areas of conflict. Psychoanalysts would see ambivalence, or lack of integration, as a relatively enduring characteristic associated with various forms of psychopathology. For example, obsessional patients cogitate at length about the positive and negative aspects of their dilemma but resist integration that would assist in minimising the conflict. The recognition of ambivalent conflicts and movement towards their resolution is a central and long-term therapeutic task. Sloan (1986) suggested that an 'ambivalent style' is the result of an individual's developmental history, and he would argue that ambivalent people experience more difficulty with all sorts of life decisions than decisive or 'unconflicted people'. Sincoff (1990) took the matter further by suggesting that varying degrees of ambivalence are present in everyone and highly ambivalent people may demonstrate a general pattern of ambivalent behaviour that is maintained by continually experiencing regret after decisions are made and reversing previous partial solutions. This decision-making style is said to be characterised by information overload and excessive self-reflection accompanied by a sense of 'self-complexity' and social sensitivity.

While ambivalence and conflict may be in part specific and inherent in the therapist/patient interaction, addiction counsellors should also perhaps look for a more general, less transient, ambivalent behavioural style in their patients. There is now a considerable body of literature that examines the characteristics of ambivalent people from a number of populations, using various measures designed to tap general ambivalence towards people and events (e.g. Raulin, 1984). By taking account of ambivalence style in treatment-resistant addicts, the therapist may be able to place this 'I want to but I do not want to change my drug-taking behaviour' dilemma in context.

The stages of change

The idea that people progress through motivational stages in their successful resolution of a problem is not new in the addiction literature (Tuchfield, 1976; Kanfer and Grimm, 1980). The stage model proposed by Prochaska and DiClemente (1984) has, however, been particularly influential (see Chapter 12). The stages of change wheel is now probably as familiar to addiction workers as Glatt's U-shaped curve. The model will not be discussed in detail here as comprehensive descriptions and critiques can be found elsewhere (DiClemente *et al.*, 1991; Davidson, 1991, 1992).

Some authors (Heather, 1992; Stockwell, 1992) have observed that the importance of the 'stage of change' model is not its detail but rather its enunciation of the 'simple truth' that a major contribution to outcome variance is the individual deciding whether or not change is in his or her best interests. The key contribution, for these authors, is the fact that the stage model places motivational interviewing in context. Stockwell (1992) would go so far as placing Miller's (1983) article on motivational interviewing at the top of any list of papers that most influenced his clinical practice. The emphasis is on dealing with motivational conflict, so it may be more apt to regard motivational interviewing as a set of ambivalence resolution strategies. The next section will examine some general principles drawn from the motivational interviewing literature that may help our patients begin to resolve their ambivalence about change.

Ambivalence resolution

Over the past decade William Miller and his colleagues have developed ideas on motivational interviewing (Miller, 1983; Miller and Rollnick, 1991; Miller and Baca, 1993) that are aimed at promoting compliance and preparedness to change. The term is, however, a misnomer, as motivational interviewing is not based on contemporary theories of the psychology of motivation. It is essentially a derivation of Rogerian client-centred counselling, and the central role of the therapist is to facilitate decision-making through clarification, advice, accurate feedback and appropriate empathy. Miller and Rollnick (1991) would argue that motivational interviewing is more task-focused and directive than traditional client-centred counselling, in that the motivational interviewer will offer advice and actively attempt to create discrepancy or dissonance, rather than passively follow the patient. However, neo-Rogerian client-centred approaches are also much more active and task orientated, with the therapist taking a less benign role than was hitherto the case (Winter, 1992). It could be argued, therefore, that motivational interviewing has adapted the psychology of self-actualisation to the treatment of addictions, but this in no way diminishes its major contribution to our understanding of change. Rollnick *et al.* (1992) say the goal of motivational interviewing is to explore ambivalence and conflicts, and to encourage patients to express their concerns and arguments about change.

As noted above, the motivational interviewer eschews the more traditional confrontational approach, which is seen as enhancing and not reducing ambivalence. The patients are instead encouraged to articulate for themselves their reasons for change rather than being directed by a coersive therapist. This is through the use of standard counselling techniques like open-ended questions, reflective listening, and affirmation. Self-motivational statements can be elicited in many ways, ranging from evocative questions to paradoxical injunction. The whole point is to develop a perceived discrepancy or dissonance between the patient's current behaviour and stated goals. Theoretically there should be a *reciprocal* relationship between dissonance and ambivalence.

With this therapeutic framework there are a number of suggested interventions that will begin to increase the likelihood of patients taking action to alter their addictive behaviour and so attenuate their motivational conflict. These include effective advice, the provision of accurate feedback, perhaps through the use of objective tests, the discussion of alternative treatment goals, the removal of practical barriers to facilitate the treatment process, and working through the decisional benefits and costs with emphasis on the positive incentives. This brief summary does not do justice to contemporary descriptions of motivational interviewing but is given as an overview of the general strategy. The approach was originally offered by Miller (1983) as a practical set of counselling strategies without any evidence for its effectiveness in reducing motivational conflict.

There have been a number of controlled trials that examine the efficacy of this type of intervention for people with alcohol problems. Like most outcome research the results give us a mixed picture. Many years ago, Ends and Page (1957) found that client-centred counselling produced greater long-term improvement when compared with other more direct interventions, and subsequent studies have confirmed that therapist empathy is a strong predictor of favourable outcome (Valle, 1981; Luborsky *et al.*, 1985). Miller and Baca (1993) found some, albeit weak, evidence of better long-term outcome in a small group of patients who received a brief motivational interview package against those who had a more direct confrontational style of intervention. Rollnick *et al.* (1992) describe a brief form of motivational intervention that is beginning to be employed to good effect in general medical settings. Conversely, in a similar setting Kuchipudi *et al.* (1990) found brief motivational interventions to be unsuccessful in altering future drinking. Baker *et al.* (1993) also found that a similar brief intervention procedure did not significantly improve HIV risk-taking behaviour among injecting drug users.

On balance it would seem likely that motivational interviewing strategies act in some way to help patients resolve ambivalence. However, further work is required to disentangle the array of elements that constitute a motivational interview and to ascertain which of these are the best predictors of future success. It seems likely that an empathic, reflective, and understanding therapist is the key variable in guiding a person towards resolution of his or her ambivalence.

Attrition

If an indicator of motivation is the probability that a person will adhere to a specific change process, then determinants of attrition from substance-abuse treatment programmes will assist our understanding of individual differences in ambivalence about treatment. Drop out rate from more formal addiction treatment programmes is not significantly different to that of other mental health treatments. For example, Garfield (1986) noted that even in private psychiatric general practice about two-thirds of patients terminate before the tenth session with the median number of sessions being around four. These figures are remarkably similar to those found by Stark (1992) in his meta analysis of 12 substance misuse drop-out studies.

Not unsurprisingly, there is a significant association between early drop out from substance-abuse treatments and poor outcome (Simpson, 1981; Walker *et al.*, 1983). Although this is a generally robust finding, there have been occasional studies that have found no such association, particularly when outcome is assessed over a long time period (Finney *et al.*, 1981). In his analysis, Stark (1992) summarises the main conclusions from this body of research. 'Length of time spent in a treatment episode' he concludes 'is moderately related to outcome for alcoholism and strongly related to outcome for drug abuse.'

A number of patient characteristics have been shown to predict drop out from substance abuse treatment programmes. There is a positive but weak relationship between variables like age, gender and social isolation, with drop out. Younger people, women, and those with limited social support, are slightly more likely prematurely to terminate treatment although this is by no means a universal finding and there is a complex interaction between gender, social factors, treatment modality and attrition. However, higher levels of pre-treatment substance use and prior treatment history are strong predictors of drop out (Beckman and Bardsley, 1986).

Of greater relevance to the present discussion is the relationship between ambivalence, expectancy and drop out. High expectations of success are associated with treatment longevity. Baekeland and Lundwall (1975) concluded that uncertainty about treatment, as assessed by clinical impression, was highly predictive of drop out. Using more direct measures of uncertainty about treatment, Rees (1985) and Noel *et al.* (1987) found, respectively, that patients who complete a pretreatment questionnaire and self-referrers are more likely to adhere to a prescribed treatment programme. It has been pointed out by both Pekarik (1985) and Garfield (1986) that patients are better able to predict eventual duration of therapy than therapists. Generally, therapists and patients disagree about the reasons for premature termination (Leigh *et al.*, 1984; Craig, 1985), with clients reporting they feel better, that they 'dislike' the therapist, or have encountered practical difficulties associated with treatment attendance. Alternatively, therapists often talk in terms of resistance or denial. Additionally, in methadone programmes patients rather than therapists invariably report that receiving methadone is more valuable than the psychotherapeutic interventions (Stark and Campbell, 1991).

Finally, there are aspects of the in-patient/out-patient treatment programmes that can enhance longevity (Chafety *et al.*, 1970; Craig, 1985; Miller, 1985; Rogalski, 1989). These include more staff, initial emphasis on concrete patient concerns, shorter waiting-lists, welcoming atmosphere, accessibility, a treatment contract, a first admission group, use of personal letters and phone calls after a missed appointment, role induction and choice of treatment. Interestingly, Rosenberg *et al.* (1976) also found that skilled female, introvert and older therapists were likely to retain patients longer.

In his review, Stark (1992) concluded that a variety of different factors promote treatment compliance, reduce treatment ambivalence, and accordingly increase the probability of change. He argued that we should see drop out as resulting from the interaction between patient needs and what the treatment service offers. Individually tailored treatment programmes that are flexible and that employ 'attrition prevention procedures' can reduce drop out and so improve outcome. Waisberg and Porter (1994) showed that an in-patient facility that acknowledged the heterogeneity of substance abusers had a dramatically lower drop out rate than one that assumed more homogeneity.

Bilsen and Emst (1989) reported an interesting combination of attrition prevention procedures and motivational interviewing strategies. What they termed Motivational Milieu Therapy (MMT) has been developed in several heroin treatment agencies in the Netherlands. Emphasis is placed on a user-friendly, safe clinical atmosphere in which trained staff initially encourage patients to discuss topics of immediate practical relevance. There are quick response times and personalised letters to patients. These are some of the simple, quality service measures noted above that can powerfully reduce attrition. In addition, MMT employs strategies drawn from the motivational interviewing literature, namely an emphasis on individal responsibility and the genuine negotiation of treatment goals between therapist and patient. While the efficacy of MMT remains to be fully established, some single case studies look promising. Of primary interest here is the combination of attrition prevention procedures and ambivalence resolution treatment strategies.

Conclusion

Much therapeutic effort with people who are trying to come to terms with an excessive behaviour is directed at encouraging persistence in the face of set-back and disappointment. The core of any intervention is the enhancement of individual motivation. There is no doubt that contemporary motivational approaches that promote positive expectation, reframing of attributions or ambivalence resolution are increasingly important weapons in the therapist's armoury. Furthermore, the work reviewed above on drop-out from treatment can help us develop more rational attrition prevention strategies so that people are more likely to adhere to a specific change process. If addiction is essentially a motivational problem then the most important challenge for all of us is to maximise goal-directed behaviour and tenacity in the use of positive change strategies.

References

Abelson, R. P. and Levi, A. (1985) Decision making and decision theory. In: Lindzey, G and Aronson, E. (eds.) *Handbook of Social Psychology*, 3rd edn, vol. 1, pp. 231–9. New York: Random House.

Annis, H. M. and Davis, C. S. (1989) Relapse prevention. In: Hester, R. K. and Miller, W. R. (eds.) *Handbook of Alcoholism Treatment Approaches: Effective Alternatives.* New York: Pergamon Press.

Baekeland, F. and Lundwall, L. (1975) Dropping out of treatment: a critical review. *Psychological Bulletin*, **82**, 738–83.

Baker, A., Heather, N., Wodak, A., Dixon, J. and Holt, P. (1993) Evaluation of a cognitive-behavioural intervention for HIV prevention among injecting drug users. *Current Science*, **7**, 247–56.

Bandura, A. (1977). *Social Learning Theory.* Englewood Cliffs, NJ: Prentice-Hall.

Bandura, A. (1985) The self and mechanisms of agency. In: Suls, J. (ed.) *Psychological Perspectives on the Self. Volume 1.* Hillsdale, NJ: Lawrence Erlbaum Associated Inc.

Beck, A. T. (1976) *Cognitive Therapy and the Emotional Disorders.* New York: International Universities Press.

Beckman, L. J. and Bardsley, P. E. (1986) Individual characteristics, gender differences, and dropout from alcoholism treatment. *Alcohol and Alcoholism*, **21**, 213–24.

Bennett, G. (1993) Improving motivation. *Addiction Counselling World*, **5**, 14–18.

Bilsen, H. van and Ernst, A. van (1989) Motivating heroin users for change. In: Bennett, G. (ed.) *Treating Drug Abusers.* London: Routledge.

Bleuler, E. (1911) *Dementia Praecox or the Group of Schizophrenias.* New York: International University Press.

Brewin, C. (1989) Cognitive change processes in psychotherapy. *Psychological Review*, **96**, 379–94.

Chaefety, M. E., Blane, H. T. and Hill, M. J. (1970) *Frontiers of Alcoholism.* New York: Science House.

Craig, R. J. (1985) Reducing the treatment dropout rate in drug abuse programmes. *Journal of Substance Abuse Treatment*, **2**, 209–19.

Davidson, R. (1991) Facilitating change in problem drinkers. In: Davidson, R., Rollnick, S. and MacEwan, I. (eds.) *Counselling Problem Drinkers.* London: Routledge.

Davidson, R. (1992) Prochaska and DiClemente's model of change: a case study. *British Journal of Addiction*, **87**, 821–22.

Davidson, R. (1994) Can psychology Make sense of change? In: Edwards, G. and Lader, M. (eds.) *Addiction: Processes of Change.* Oxford: Oxford University Press.

Davies, J. B. (1992) *The Myth of Addiction.* Reading: Harwood Academic.

Davies, P. (1981) Expectations and therapeutic practices in out-patient clinics for alcohol problems. *British Journal of Addiction*, **76**, 159–73.

DiClemente, C. C., Prochaska, J. O., Fairhurst, S. K., Velicer, W. F., Velasquex, M. M. and Rossi, J. S. (1991) The processes of smoking cessation: an analysis of precontemplation, contemplation, and preparation stages of change. *Journal of Consulting and Clinical Psychology*, **59**, 295–304.

Dobson, K. S. (1988) *Handbook of Cognitive-Behavioural Therapies*. New York: Guilford Press.

Dollard, J. and Miller, N. E. (1950) *Personality and Psychotherapy*. New York: McGraw-Hill.

Ends, E. J. and Page, C. W. (1957) A study of three types of group psychotherapy with hospitalized male inebriates. *Quarterly Journal of Studies on Alcohol*, **18**, 263–77.

Festinger, L. (1957) *A Theory of Cognitive Dissonance*. Evanston, IL: Row, Peterson.

Finney, J., Moos, R. and Chan, D. (1981) Length of stay and programme component effects in the treatment of alcoholism: a comparison of two techniques for process analysis. *Journal of Consulting and Clinical Psychology*, **49**, 120–31.

Frankl, V. (1969) *The Will to Meaning: Foundations and Applications of Logotherapy*. New York: New American Library.

Freud, S. (1913) Totem and taboo. In: Strachey, J. (ed.) *The Standard Edition of the Complete Psychological Works of Sigmund Freud*, vol. 14, pp. 243–58. London: Hogarth.

Garfield, S. L. (1986) Research on client variables in psychotherapy. In: Garfield, S. L. and Bergin, A. E. (eds.) *Handbook of Psychotherapy and Behaviour Change*, 3rd edn, pp. 213–56. New York: Wiley.

Heather, N. (1992) Addictive disorders are essentially motivational problems. *British Journal of Addiction*, **87**, 828–30.

Heider, F. (1958) *The Psychology of Interpersonal Relations*. New York: Wiley.

Holder, A. (1975) Theoretical and clinical aspects of ambivalence. *Psychoanalytic Study of the Child*, **30**, 197–220.

Hull, C. (1943) *Principles of Behaviour*. New York: Appleton-Century-Crofts.

Janis, I. and Mann, L. (1977) *Decision-making: A Psychological Analysis of Conflict, Choice and Commitment*. New York: Free Press.

Kanfer, F. H. and Grimm, G. L. (1980) Managing clinical change: a process model of therapy. *Behaviour Modification*, **4**, 419–44.

Kuchipudi, V., Hobein, K., Fleckinger, A. and Iber, F. L. (1990) Failure of a two-hour motivational intervention to alter recurrent drinking behaviour in alcoholics with gastrointestinal disease. *Journal of Studies on Alcohol*, **51**, 356–60.

Leake, G. J. and King, A. S. (1977) Effect of counsellor expectations on alcohol recovery. *Alcohol Health and Research World*, **11**, 16–22.

Leigh, B. C. (1989) In search of the seven dwarves: issues of measurement and meaning in alcohol expectancy research. *Psychological Bulletin*, **105**(3), 361–73.

Leigh, G., Osborne, A. C. and Cleland, P. (1984) Factors associated with patient dropout from an outpatient alcoholism treatment service. *Journal of Studies on Alcohol*, **45**, 359–62.

Lewin, K. (1947) Frontiers in group dynamics: concept, method and reality in social equilibrium and social change. *Human Relations*, **6**, 5–41.

Lick, J. and Bootzin, R. (1975) Expectancy factors in the treatment of fear: methodological and theoretical issues. *Psychological Bulletin*, **82**, 917–31.

Luborsky, L., McLellan, A. T., Woody, G. E., O'Brien, C. P. and Auerbach, A. (1985) Therapist success and its determinants. *Archives of General Psychiatry*, **42**, 602–11.

Marlatt, G. A. and Gordon, J. R. (1985) *Relapse Prevention: Maintenance Strategies in the Treatment of Addictive Behaviour.* New York: Guilford Press.

Miller, W. R. (1983) Motivational interviewing with problem drinkers. *Behavioural Psychotherapy*, **11**, 147–72.

Miller, W. R. (1985) Motivation for treatment: a review with special emphasis on alcoholism. *Psychological Bulletin*, **98**, 84–107.

Miller, W. R. and Baca, L. M. (1993) Two year follow-up of bibliotherapy and therapist-directed controlled drinking training for problem drinkers. *Behaviour Therapy*, **14**, 441–8.

Miller, W. and Rollnick, S. (1991) *Motivational interviewing: preparing people to change addictive behaviour.* New York: Guilford.

McClelland, D. C. (1961) *The Achieving Society.* New York: Free Press.

Newcomb, M. and Harlow, L. (1986) Life events and substance use among adolescents: Mediating effects of perceived loss of control and meaninglessness in life. *Journal of Personality and Social Psychology*, **51**, 564–77.

Noel, N. E., McCrady, B. S., Stout, R. L. and Fisher-Nelson, H. (1987) Predictors of attrition from an outpatient alcoholism treatment programme for couples. *Journal of Studies on Alcohol*, **3**, 229–35.

Pekarik, G. (1985) Coping with dropouts. *Professional Psychology: Research and Practice*, **16**, 114–23.

Prochaska, J. O. and DiClemente, C. C. (1984) *The Transtheoretical Approach: Crossing Traditional Boundaries of Therapy.* New York: Dow-Jones Irwin.

Raulin, M. L. (1984) Development of a scale to measure intense ambivalence. *Journal of Consulting and Clinical Psychology*, **52**, 53–72.

Rees, D. W. (1985) Health beliefs and compliance with alcoholism treatment. *Journal of Studies on Alcohol*, **46**, 517–24.

Rogalski, C. J. (1989) Attrition within a detoxification unit: patient response to policy and psychological intervention. *The International Journal of the Addictions*, **24**, 279–301.

Rollnik, S., Heather, N. and Bell, A. (1992) Negotiating behaviour change in medical settings: The development of brief motivational interviewing. *Journal of Mental Health*, **1**, 25–37.

Rosenberg, C. M., Gerrein, J. R., Manohar, V. and Liftik, J. (1976) Evaluation of training of alcoholism counselors. *Journal of Studies on Alcohol*, **37**, 1236–46.

Rotter, J. B. (1975) Some problems and misconceptions related to the construct of internal versus external control of reinforcement. *Journal of Consulting and Clinical Psychology*, **43**, 56–67.

Russell, M., Armstrong, E. and Patel, U. (1976) Temporal continuity in electric aversion therapy for cigarette smoking. *Behaviour Research and Therapy*, **14**, 103–23.

Simpson, D. D. (1981) Treatment for drug abuse: follow-up outcomes and length of time spent. *Archives of General Psychiatry*, **38**, 875–80.

Sincoff, J. (1990) The psychological characteristics of ambivalent people. *Clinical Psychology Review*, **10**, 43–68.

Sloan, T. S. (1986) *Deciding: Self-deception in Life Choices.* New York: Methuen.

Stark, M. (1992) Dropping out of substance abuse treatment. A clinically oriented review. *Clinical Psychology Review*, **12**, 93–116.

Stark, M. J. and Campbell, B. K. (1991) A psychoeducational approach to methadone maintenance treatment: a survey of client reactions. *Journal of Substance Abuse Treatment*, **8**, 125–31.

Stockwell, T. (1992) Models of change, heavenly bodies and weltanschauungs. *British Journal of Addiction*, **87**, 830–1.

Tolman, E. C. (1948) Cognitive maps in rats and men. *Psychological Review*, **55**, 189–208.

Tuchfield, B. (1976) *Changes in the Patterns of Alcohol Use Without the Aid of Formal Treatment*. North Carolina: Research Triangle Institute.

Valle, S. K. (1981) Interpersonal functioning of alcoholism counsellors and treatment outcome. *Journal of Studies on Alcohol*, **42**, 783–90.

Wade, C. and Tarvis, C. (1993) *Psychology*. New York: Harper Collins.

Waisberg, J. and Porter, J. (1994) Purpose of life and outcome of treatment for alcohol dependence. *British Journal of Clinical Psychology*, **33**, 49–64.

Walker, R. D., Donovan, D. M., Kivlahan, D. R. and O'Leary, M. R. (1983) Length of stay, neuropsychological performance and aftercare: influences on alcohol treatment outcome. *Journal of Consulting and Clinical Psychology*, **51**, 900–11.

Weiner, B. (1985) An attributional theory of achievement motivation and emotion. *Psychological Review*, **92**, 548–73.

Winter, D. (1992) *Personal Construct Psychology in Clinical Practice*. London: Routledge.

12

Can 'stages of change' provide guidance in the treatment of addictions? A critical examination of Prochaska and DiClemente's model

STEPHEN SUTTON

Introduction

Few workers in the addictions field can fail to have noticed the 'stages of change' model of Prochaska and DiClemente (Prochaska and DiClemente, 1986; Prochaska *et al.*, 1992). The model appears to offer a general, comprehensive, and theoretically coherent account of how people change their behaviour. It clearly has immense intuitive appeal to teachers, practitioners and researchers in the addictions field. With one exception (Davidson, 1992), commentators have been unanimous in their praise and enthusiasm for the model. Orford (1992) likened the development of the model to a Kuhnian paradigm shift, and Stockwell (1992) compared the reaction of some of his colleagues to the recent announcement that a fifth stage of change had been identified to the awe that might accompany the discovery of a new planet.

This chapter provides a critical assessment of the stages of change model. It addresses two key assumptions of the model: (1) that change in addictive behaviour involves movement through a sequence of stages; and (2) that different processes of change are emphasised in different stages and promote progression through the sequence. The questionnaire instruments designed to assess the stages and processes of change are also examined. The chapter does not attempt to give an exhaustive review of the literature in this area. It focuses on Prochaska and DiClemente's own published papers. Related work on readiness to change (Rollnick *et al.*, 1992; Heather *et al.*, 1993) is not discussed, though some of the comments also apply to that approach. Nor do we compare the stages of change model with other decision-making models that have been applied to addictive behaviours such as the Theory of Reasoned Action/Planned Behaviour and the Subjective Expected Utility Model (Sutton, 1987, 1989). Most applications of the stages of change model have been to smoking. Orford (1992) has suggested that decision-making approaches may be less applicable to alcohol and drug abuse.

The stages of change
The stages of change model

The stages of change have been described in terms of a revolving door metaphor, as depicted in Figure 12.1. As an aside, it is worth noting that the metaphor is not strictly accurate since a person entering a revolving door stays in the same compartment ('stage') until exiting. The first stage is **precontemplation** (not seriously thinking about changing). The circle of change is entered by the **contemplation** stage in which the individual starts to think seriously about changing his or her behaviour. In the model, the contemplation stage is followed by the **action** stage in which the individual makes an attempt to quit. Successful individuals will enter the **maintenance** stage and may eventually reach termination. (Termination is not yet officially recognised as one of the stages of

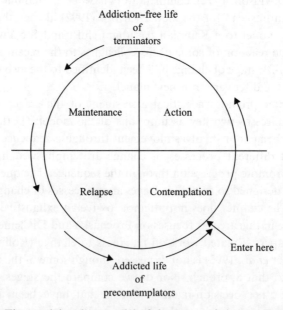

Figure 12.1 The revolving-door model of the stages of change. From Prochaska and DiClemente (1986), p. 6. Copyright 1986 by Plenum Press. Reproduced with permission.

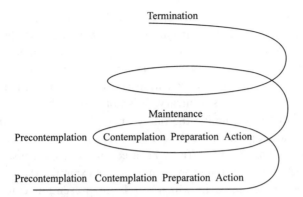

Figure 12.2 A spiral model of the stages of change. From Prochaska *et al.* (1992), p. 1104. Copyright 1992 by the American Psychological Association. Reproduced with permission.

change.) More likely, however, he or she will **relapse**, and will typically cycle through the stages several times before achieving long-term maintenance.

Prochaska *et al.* (1992) have recently presented a spiral model, which they say more accurately illustrates how most people move through the stages of change (Figure 12.2). Unlike the revolving door model, this model allows an individual to cycle back to precontemplation more than once before eventually achieving termination of the problem. The preparation stage has recently been added between contemplation and action. People in this stage are described as being 'ready for action'. Relapse is no longer regarded as a stage of change but rather as an event that marks the end of the action or maintenance stage.

Prochaska and DiClemente have used two different methods for assessing the stages of change: a simple categorisation based on three or four questionnaire items (what they call a 'staging algorithm') and a Stages of Change Questionnaire, which yields scale scores on each of four dimensions corresponding to the different stages. To my knowledge, these two methods have never been used together in the same study. Thus there are no data available on how well they agree. Nor is there much evidence on whether they yield consistent results when related to other measures.

Categorical definition of stages

Table 12.1 shows an example of a categorical definition of stages (based on that used by DiClemente *et al.* 1991 in their study of smoking cessation). This definition divides users (smokers, drinkers, drug users) and ex-users into five mutually exclusive and exhaustive categories. The first three categories contain the current users, the remaining two the ex-users. The definition defines stages in such a way that maintenance can only follow action, i.e. the only way of reaching the maintenance stage is by way of the action stage. The transition between action and maintenance can be measured but it is arbitrary. It is not marked by an event of any personal significance, unlike the one-year anniversary of starting a successful quit attempt might be. There is no reason to expect that different processes of change will start to be used simply as a consequence of passing the six-month milestone – unless, for example, the person is in a treatment programme in which a relapse prevention component is introduced at this point.

Although the transition from the action to the maintenance 'stage' is arbitrary, entry into the action stage itself is marked, at least in a cold-turkey quitter, by a discrete and observable shift from using to non-using. The movement from precontemplation to contemplation can also be thought of as a true stage transition, albeit one that is not directly observable, in that the person shifts from a state of not seriously thinking about quitting to a state in which he or she is seriously thinking about quitting. (Even so, we would not expect someone in the contemplation stage to be *constantly* thinking about quitting.)

A further problem with the scheme in Table 12.1 is that users can only be in the preparation stage if they have made a recent quit attempt. It follows that first-time quitters can never have been in the preparation stage at any time in their using history.

Table 12.1 *Categorical definition of stages*

Precontemplation (PC)
Currently using and not seriously considering quitting within the next 6 months

Contemplation (C)
Currently using and seriously considering quitting within the next 6 months but either (1) not planning to quit within the next 30 days or (2) has not made at least one 24-hour quit attempt in the past year, or both

Preparation (PA)
Currently using, seriously considering quitting within the next 6 months, planning to quit within the next 30 days, and has made at least one 24-hour quit attempt in the past year

Action (A)
Currently not using; quit in the last 6 months

Maintenance (M)
Currently not using; quit > 6 months ago

The categorical definition essentially divides users into three groups based on their *intention* to quit (with the added complication that recent quit attempts are also taken into account). Other decision-making models employ a continuous measure of intention. In these 'continuum' models, the strength of intention to quit is assumed to fluctuate over time within individuals but there is no necessary assumption that the change is monotonic or that it involves crossing a sequence of thresholds. Thus the stages of change model can be regarded as imposing an artificial categorisation and ordering on what may actually be an underlying continuous process. Even so, such a categorisation may serve a useful purpose, just as dividing people into introverts and extroverts may be useful for some purposes.

The Stages of Change Scales

An alternative to the categorical definition of stages is the Stages of Change Questionnaire (also known by the acronym URICA – University of Rhode Island Change Assessment). This consists of 32 items, eight for each of the four stages (the preparation stage is not represented). Table 12.2 gives sample items. The items refer generically to the subject's 'problem' but do not specify a particular problem behaviour. The scales seem more appropriate to clinical settings than to self-change. Some items seem to be tapping motivation to come for treatment. For example, if someone agrees with the statement 'I am finally

Table 12.2 *The Stages of Change Scales (URICA): sample items*

Precontemplation
'As far as I'm concerned, I don't have any problems that need changing'
'All this talk about psychology is boring. Why can't people just forget about their problems?'

Contemplation
'I have a problem and I really think I should work on it'
'I'm hoping this place will help me to better understand myself'

Action
'I am doing something about the problems that had been bothering me'
'Anyone can talk about change: I'm actually doing something about it'

Maintenance
'It worries me that I might slip back on a problem I have already changed, so I am here to seek help'
'I'm here to prevent myself from having a relapse of my problem'

---

doing something about the problems that had been bothering me' (an action item), they may be referring to their decision to come for treatment rather than their decision to change their problem behaviour; these are not necessarily the same.

To obtain information on reliability and validity, the questionnaire was administered to two separate clinical samples (McConnaughy *et al.*, 1983; McConnaughy *et al.*, 1989). In each case, factor analysis (principal components) yielded a similar four-factor solution.This is what would be expected given that the questionnaire was designed to assess four separate dimensions. Four scale scores were calculated for each subject by adding up his or her scores on the eight items making up those scales, and Pearson product-moment correlations among the scales were computed. The highest correlations were between adjacent stages. Thus, the contemplation and action scales correlated around 0.50, as did the action and maintenance scales. In other words, there was a tendency for subjects who scored highly on contemplation also to score highly on action; similarly, for action and maintenance. A pattern in which adjacent stages are more highly correlated than other pairs of stages is known as a simplex pattern. The researchers interpreted this as evidence supporting the stages of change model.

There are a number of problems wth this interpretation. First, particularly in the 1989 sample, the correlation between the contemplation and maintenance scales, representing non-adjacent stages, was almost as large as – and probably not significantly different from – the correlations between adjacent stages. In a small study of drug users, Abellanas and McLellan (1993) also found high correlations between non-adjacent stages. Second, the correlation between precontemplation and contemplation was *negative* (around -0.50 in each sample). As would be predicted, subjects who had high scores on precontemplation tended to have low scores on contemplation. The problem for the stages of change model is that it cannot be supported by a pattern of correlations in which some correlations between consecutive stages are positive and others are negative.

The data in fact argue against a stage model. They indicate that it is possible, indeed common, for someone to have an above-average score on two or more 'stages' simultaneously. This was confirmed in both the McConnaughy *et al.* studies by the results of cluster analyses conducted with the aim of identifying a small number of distinct client profiles. In the more recent paper, the authors presented an eight-cluster solution. Several of the clusters were characterised by profiles of above-average scores on two or more stages. For example, the 44 subjects in the 'Decision-making' cluster were characterised by a profile of below-average scores on precontemplation and maintenance, and above-average scores on contemplation and action. These subjects can be thought of as being in two different stages at once. If this interpretation is accepted, the concept of stage loses its meaning.

A version of the Stages of Change Scales called SOCRATES (Stages of Change Readiness and Treatment Eagerness Scale), which is specific to alcohol and drug abuse, has been developed by Miller and colleagues in the United States (W. R. Miller, 1993, personal communication), but no published applications have so far appeared.

Movement through the stages

The concept of stage implies ordering or sequence. Someone in a given stage is assumed to have come from the preceding stage in the sequence and to be on the way to the next stage. Several studies have assessed subjects (smokers and ex-smokers) on two or more occasions enabling movement between stages to be examined. Prochaska *et al.* (1991) reported data on a sample of 544 self-changers (out of an initial sample of 960), who provided information about stage of change every six months for two years. Although this study suffered from the problem of attrition frequently encountered in longitudinal studies, it is nevertheless an important and unusual dataset. The patterns of movement through the stages are not reported completely but it is possible to extract some key findings from the paper. In particular, only 16% of subjects showed a stable progression over the two years from one stage to the next in the sequence (e.g. precontemplation to contemplation) without suffering any reverses, e.g. PC–PC–PC–C–C. There were apparently no subjects who showed a stable progression through three or more stages (e.g. PC–PC–C–C–A); two was the maximum. Twelve per cent of subjects moved backwards one or two stages (e.g. C–C–C–PC–PC). Thirty-six per cent of subjects showed a flat profile, that is they stayed in the same stage across the five waves of measurement (e.g. PC–PC–PC–PC–PC).

This study in effect took five 'snapshots' over a two-year period. It is quite possible that many subjects moved through other stages in the six-month periods between measurements. The study did not attempt to find out what went on between follow-ups; only the subject's current stage was recorded. With this caveat, the findings as reported show clearly that forward progressive movement through the stages is far from being the modal pattern of change among volunteer self-changers.

Further studies of this kind need to be conducted in different subject samples (e.g. problem drinkers identified in primary care settings, heroin users in methadone maintenance programmes). Subjects entering formal treatment programmes will be more homogeneous than self-changers in the community. For one thing, except in relapse prevention programmes, one would not expect to find any maintainers at start of treatment, though there may be a few recent quitters. It is possible that in such settings movement between stages will be more systematic and more consistent with the sequence postulated by the model. Relevant data have been reported by DiClemente *et al.* (1991). Smokers participating in a self-help cessation programme were divided into precontemplators, contemplators, and those who were prepared for action. Stage of change at baseline predicted the probability of attempting to quit as well as smoking status at one and six months (i.e. movement to the action stage). This is consistent with a number of studies showing that current intentions to quit and past behaviour (prior quit attempts) predict the probability of making an attempt to quit (e.g. Sutton, 1989; Sutton *et al.*, 1987).

In any longitudinal study, adherence to the sequence of stages implied by the stages of change model can be analysed 'prospectively', by calculating the chances of moving from a given stage to the next stage in the sequence, or 'retrospectively', by calculating the probability of coming from the preceding stage. The predictions of the model could be formalised in these terms. For example, precontemplators, if they change at all, should be most likely to move to the contemplation stage. And those who are in the contemplation stage, if they have moved from another stage, should be most likely to have come from the precontemplation stage.

One difficulty with the model that has a bearing on all such analyses is that it says nothing about how long people stay in a particular stage or when, and under what circumstances, they change stages (except in the trivial case of movement between action and maintenance). The stages of change model is thus not, as is sometimes claimed, a model that describes *when* people change.

States of change

It may be more useful to think in terms of *states* of change rather than stages of change. Unlike stages, states carry no implication of ordering or

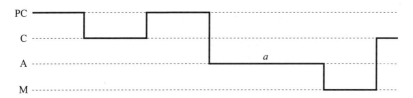

Figure 12.3 Timeline showing one individual's movement between different states of change. (PC = Precontemplation, C = Contemplation, A = Action, M = Maintenance.)

sequence. Figure 12.3 shows a timeline representing one hypothetical individual's movement between different states. The states are given the same names as Prochaska and DiClemente's stages. The horizontal axis represents time. The length of a horizontal line represents the duration of time spent in that state. The maximum length of line *a* is fixed by the definition of action (e.g. six months). This particular individual starts off in the precontemplation state, then has a spell in contemplation before moving back to precontemplation. He or she then decides to quit smoking and succeeds in doing so for at least six months before relapsing and moving to the contemplation state. The bridge on the rightmost vertical line indicates that the action state is bypassed: the individual moves straight from maintenance to contemplation without going through any intermediate state. If information is available on such durations in a sample of individuals, event history methods (an extension of survival analysis) can be used to analyse the factors associated with transitions between states.

The processes of change

The second core dimension of the model is the processes of change. Initially through analysing a large number of different systems of therapy, Prochaska and DiClemente identified ten processes of change. These are covert or overt activities that people engage in to help them progress towards recovery. They are assumed to be common to self-change and to change that occurs within a formal treatment programme. The processes are listed in Table 12.3 along with a brief description. In Prochaska and DiClemente's model, the processes of change are integrated with the stages of change in the sense that different processes are assumed to be emphasised in different stages.

The Processes of Change Questionnaire

A 40-item questionnaire designed to assess ten basic processes of change was developed using a large sample of smokers and ex-smokers who responded to newspaper reports and advertisements (Prochaska *et al.*, 1988). Table 12.3 gives sample items. The response format used in most applications asks the respondent to rate the frequency of use of each process in the last month on a five-point scale from 1 = *never* to 5 = *repeatedly*.

Table 12.3 *Labels, definitions, and sample questionnaire items for the Ten Processes of Change*

Consciousness raising: Increasing information about self and problem
    'I recall articles dealing with the problem of quitting smoking'

Self-liberation: Choosing and commitment to act or belief in ability to change
    'I tell myself I can choose to smoke or not'

Dramatic relief: Experiencing and expressing feelings about one's problems and solutions
    'Warnings about health hazards of smoking move me emotionally'

Environmental reevaluation: Assessing how one's problem affects physical environment
    'I stop to think that smoking is polluting the environment'

Helping relationships: Being open and trusting about problems with someone who cares
    'Special people in my life accept me the same whether I smoke or not'

Stimulus control: Avoiding or countering stimuli that elicit problem behaviours
    'I remove things from my home that remind me of smoking'

Counter-conditioning: Substituting alternatives for problem behaviours
    'Instead of smoking, I engage in some physical activity'

Social liberation: Increasing alternatives for non-problem behaviours available in society
    'I notice that public places have sections set aside for smoking'

Self-reevaluation: Assessing how one feels and thinks about oneself with respect to a problem
    'My dependency on cigarettes makes me feel disappointment in myself'

Reinforcement management: Rewarding oneself or being rewarded by others for making changes
    'I can expect to be rewarded by others if I don't smoke'

All the items are framed positively; they are all intended to represent activities that help smokers to move through the stages. Processes that may hinder movement towards smoking cessation (e.g. activities that operate to keep individuals in the contemplation stage or that promote regression to an earlier stage) are not represented in the questionnaire. Examples of such negative processes might be procrastination, avoidance, wishful thinking, minimisation of the problem, self-attribution of addiction (see Eiser *et al.*, 1978), self-blame, and 'reactance' aroused by other people's attempts to persuade one to change. From the standpoint of the model, these processes would be regarded as maladaptive, though they may have beneficial effects on psychological well-being.

Some items on the questionnaire reflect passive rather than active processes, for example, 'I am rewarded by others if I don't smoke'. Some items seem to reflect static conditions rather than dynamic processes, for example, 'I have someone who listens when I need to talk about my smoking'.

A key hypothesis in the stages of change model is that different processes will be used in different stages. In a cross-sectional study of smokers and ex-smokers, Prochaska and DiClemente (1983) found significant differences in the processes used across stages; these are summarised in Table 12.4. Not surprisingly, precontemplators reported using eight of the ten processes less frequently than the other groups. Again not

Table 12.4 *Processes of change listed under the stages in which they are emphasised most and least*

Precontemplation	$\longrightarrow$	Contemplation	$\longrightarrow$	Action	$\longrightarrow$	Maintenance
Eight processes used the least		Consciousness raising				
			Self-reevaluation[a]			
			Self-liberation			
			Helping relationship			
			Reinforcement management			
				Counter-conditioning[a]		
				Stimulus control[a]		

[a]Processes emphasised in two stages are shown overlapping both stages.
From Prochaska and DiClemente (1983), p. 394. Copyright 1983 by the American Psychological Association, adapted by permission.

surprisingly, behavioural processes tended to be used more frequently in the action and maintenance stages (i.e. by those who had stopped smoking). Some processes seemed to be emphasised in two consecutive stages. For example, counterconditioning (substituting other activities or thoughts for smoking) and stimulus control (removing reminders of smoking) were used more than average in both action and maintenance. Prochaska and DiClemente interpret this as indicating that these processes bridge the two stages and as supporting the idea that engaging in these processes will help to move the individual from action to maintenance.

This interpretation is problematic, and the problem is exacerbated by the cross-sectional design of the study. To the extent that two stages do not differ with respect to the frequency with which particular processes of change are used, then this is evidence against making a distinction between them. If, on the other hand, a given process is emphasised in one stage but not in the next, how can we tell whether this is helping or hindering movement across stages? For example, people in the contemplation stage appeared to have been engaging in consciousness raising more frequently in the previous month than people in other stages. But thinking about stopping smoking could be a substitute for action rather than a step towards it. It would be useful to have information on how long a person has been in that stage. If a smoker has been in the contemplation stage for two years and is still raising his or her consciousness about stopping smoking, this would seem to suggest that this process is not helping them move towards making an attempt to quit.

The processes of change appear to have some predictive value. Prochaska *et al.* (1985) reported the results of discriminant function analyses predicting movement between stages over a six-month period in a large sample of smokers and ex-smokers. All but one of the ten processes (environmental re-evaluation) occurred in one or more of the six discriminant functions (prediction equations) that emerged from the analysis. However, more frequent use of a process was sometimes predictive of progression to a more advanced stage and sometimes predictive of no movement or regression to an earlier stage; positive and negative predictive relationships occurred with about equal frequency. For example, one discriminant function distinguished contemplators who became precontemplators from those who became recent quitters. The latter group was relatively high in self-re-evaluation but relatively *low* in consciousness raising. A second discriminant function distinguished contemplators who became recent quitters from those who stayed in the contemplation stage. Those who took action were those who had been low in self-re-evaluation and low in social liberation.

It is difficult to draw any clear recommendations for treatment or self-change from these results. Contemplators would have to be advised not to use consciousness raising or social liberation because these processes appear to be counterproductive for people at their stage. Self-re-evaluation may or may not be helpful. The remaining processes were unrelated to progression.

The findings of this study also show some clear discrepancies with those of Prochaska and DiClemente (1983). For example, in that study, consciousness raising was emphasised in the contemplation stage. But in the Prochaska *et al.* (1985) paper, greater frequency of use of consciousness raising appeared to have an adverse effect. In the 1983 paper, reinforcement management was used most frequently in the action stage. In the 1985 paper, this process occurred in only one discriminant function (for the precontemplators) and did not have a large weight. Several other important inconsistencies between the two sets of results could be cited.

Processes of change over a two-year period

Prochaska *et al.* (1991) assessed the processes of change every six months over a two-year period in their sample of self-changers. They reported the results separately for each process using graphs like that shown in Figure 12.4 for self-re-evaluation. The graph is constructed by placing the following six subgroups end to end: those who stayed in precontemplation throughout the two-year period; those who moved from precontemplation to contemplation; those who moved from contemplation to action; those who stayed in the action stage; those who moved from action to maintenance; and those who stayed in maintenance. There was a total of 260 subjects in these six subgroups, representing 48% of those who provided complete information across all five waves and 27% of the initial sample. These subgroups were selected with the aim of identifying patterns of successful change. At each wave, those who had quit smoking but then relapsed were assigned to contemplation.

With the exception of social liberation, the processes tended to be used most frequently by individuals in one or more of the inner groups (those who progressed from contemplation to action, or stayed in the action stage, or progressed from action to maintenance) and least frequently by the outer groups (those who stayed in precontemplation, progressed from precontemplation to contemplation, or stayed in maintenance).

202   *Stephen Sutton*

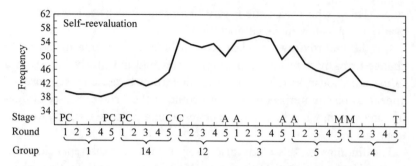

Figure 12.4 Frequency of use (T scores) of self-reevaluation by six profile groups integrated across four stages of change. From Prochaska and DiClemente (1986), p. 14. Copyright 1986 by Plenum Press. Reproduced with permission.

The authors discuss the results in terms of mountain metaphor (*Mt. Change*). 'The change processes followed a general curvilinear pattern of *climbing* from precontemplation to contemplation, *peaking* at a particular stage of change, and then *descending* either to precontemplation levels or to somewhat higher levels if used as relapse prevention strategies during the maintenance stage' (Prochaska *et al.* 1991, p. 102). They argue that the point at which different processes peak can be useful in developing interventions. For example, consciousness raising peaks during contemplation, suggesting that the processing of information about smoking and quitting is a central process for the contemplation stage.

However, although the cross-sequential methodology used by Prochaska and colleagues is an interesting way of depicting patterns of change, it does not directly address the question of whether the use of a particular process of change helped individuals in a particular stage to progress over the two years. What we really need to know, for example, is whether contemplators who moved to the action stage employed particular processes of change more or less frequently than contemplators who made no progress; it is not possible to extract this information from the graphs since the latter subgroup is not represented. Furthermore, no significance tests are reported so it is not possible to gauge whether the greater use of some processes by subjects in some subgroups reflects a real difference. In connection with this, it should be noted that the sample sizes for some of the subgroups were small; there were only 14 individuals who progressed from precontemplation to contemplation and only 17 who moved from contemplation to action.

Stage-matched interventions

One attraction of a stage model is that it suggests the possibility of stage-matched interventions in which subjects in different stages of change receive different versions of an intervention package rather than the same standardised package. Prochaska and colleagues (Prochaska *et al.*, 1993; Velicer *et al.*, 1993) developed stage-based self-help smoking cessation manuals and tested them in a randomised controlled study against existing manuals. Participants in the 'individualised manual' condition were sent the manual matched to their individual stage of change and manuals for all the subsequent stages. Using a criterion of prolonged abstinence, there was no significant advantage for the individualised manuals. Abstinence rates were around 3% at 12 months and 7% and 5% at 18 months in the stage-matched and standardised conditions respectively. Other conditions involving repeated contact with participants roughly doubled these success rates. Given the evidence concerning processes of change summarised above, it is not surprising that the individualised manuals were not more effective than the best available self-help manuals. To my knowledge, no controlled studies of stage-matched intervention programmes for problem drinkers or drug users have yet been published.

Conclusions

We need models of change to clarify our thinking, to integrate research findings, to generate new hypotheses and to guide clinical practice. The stages of change model has intuitive appeal and heuristic value. This chapter has examined the evidence for two key assumptions of the model. Contrary to the model, there is no strong evidence that using particular processes in particular stages promotes movement to subsequent stages, and hence little reason to expect stage-matched interventions that encourage the use of these processes to be particularly effective. Moreover, outside treatment and intervention settings, people do not move through the stages of change in an ordered fashion. Nor do they cycle through the stages in the way that the spiral representation of the model suggests. Motivation or intention to change may be more realistically thought of as a continuum with no necessary assumption that people move along this continuum in one direction or through a sequence of discrete stages. On this view, imposing a discrete categorisation may be convenient for some purposes as long as it is recognised that the categorisation is an artificial one – it is misleading to speak of 'discovering' a new stage – and that movement along the continuum, or through the categories, may not involve an invariant temporal sequence. Even if it is argued that the stage categorisation is not artificial in this sense, then it still may be more appropriate to think in terms of states of change rather than stages of change; stages imply sequence whereas states do not.

The stages of change model is not an accurate description of how people change. It should be thought of not as a descriptive model but as a *prescriptive* model – a model of *ideal* change. It prescribes how, from the viewpoint of a therapist or a health educator, people *should* change and suggests how they might be encouraged or helped to change. As such, it may be useful in designing interventions. If people can be persuaded to change in accordance with the logical sequence implied by the model (e.g. thinking about something for a time before doing it), then the stages of change model may yet contribute to the development of more effective programmes.

References

Abellanas, L. and McLellan, T. (1993) 'Stage of Change' by drug problem in concurrent opioid, cocaine, and cigarette users. *Journal of Psychoactive Drugs*, **25**, 307–13.

Davidson, R. (1992) Prochaska and DiClemente's model of change: a case study? *British Journal of Addiction*, **87**, 821–2.

DiClemente, C. C., Prochaska, J. O., Fairhurst, S. K.,Velicer, W. F., Velasquez, M. M. and Rossi, J. R. (1991) The process of smoking cessation: an analysis of precontemplation, contemplation, and preparation stages of change. *Journal of Consulting and Clinical Psychology*, **59**, 295–304.

Eiser, J. R., Sutton, S. R. and Wober, M. (1978) 'Consonant' and 'dissonant' smokers and the self-attribution of addiction. *Addictive Behaviors*, **3**, 99–106.

Heather, N., Rollnick, S. and Bell, A. (1993) Predictive validity of the Readiness to Change Questionnaire. *Addiction*, **88**, 1667–77.

McConnaughy, E. A., DiClemente, C. C., Prochaska, J. O. and Velicer, W. (1989) Stages of change in psychotherapy: a follow-up report. *Psychotherapy*, **26**, 494–503.

McConnaughy, E. A., Prochaska, J. O. and Velicer, W. F. (1983) Stages of change in psychotherapy: measurement and sample profiles. *Psychotherapy: Theory, Research and Practice*, **20**, 368–75.

Orford, J. (1992) Davidson's dilemma. *British Journal of Addiction*, **88**, 832–33.

Prochaska, J. O. and DiClemente, C. C. (1983) Stages and processes of self-change of smoking: toward an integrative model of change. *Journal of Consulting and Clinical Psychology*, **51**, 390–5.

Prochaska, J. O. and DiClemente, C. C. (1986) Toward a comprehensive model of change. In: Miller, W. R. and Heather, N. (eds.) *Treating addictive behaviors: processes of change*, pp. 3–27. New York: Plenum.

Prochaska, J. O., DiClemente, C. C. and Norcross, J. C. (1992) In search of how people change: applications to addictive behaviors. *American Psychologist*, **7**, 1102–14.

Prochaska, J. O., DiClemente, C. C., Velicer, W., Ginpil, S. and Norcross, J. C. (1985) Predicting change in smoking status for self-changers. *Addictive Behaviors*, **10**, 395–406.

Prochaska, J. O., DiClemente, C. C.,Velicer, W. and Rossi, J. S. (1993) Standardized, individualized, interactive, and personalized self-help programs for smoking cessation. *Health Psychology*, **12**, 399–405.

Prochaska, J. O., Velicer, W., DiClemente, C. C. and Fava, J. (1988) Measuring processes of change: applications to the cessation of smoking. *Journal of Consulting and Clinical Psychology*, **56**, 520–8.

Prochaska, J. O., Velicer, W., Guadagnoli, E., Rossi, J. S. and DiClemente, C. C. (1991) Patterns of change: dynamic typology applied to smoking cessation. *Multivariate Behavioral Research*, **26**, 83–107.

Rollnick, S., Heather, N., Gold, R. and Hall, W. (1992) Development of a short 'readiness to change' questionnaire for use in brief, opportunistic interventions among excessive drinkers. *British Journal of Addiction*, **87**, 743–54.

Stockwell, T. (1992) Models of change, heavenly bodies and weltanschauungs. *British Journal of Addiction*, **88**, 830–2.

Sutton, S. R. (1987) Social-psychological approaches to understanding addictive behaviours: attitude-behaviour and decision-making models. *British Journal of Addiction*, **82**, 355–70.

Sutton, S. R. (1989) Smoking attitudes and behavior: Applications of Fishbein and Ajzen's theory of reasoned action to predicting and understanding smoking decisions. In: Ney, T. and Gale, A. (eds.) *Smoking and human behavior*, pp. 289–312. Chichester: Wiley.

Sutton, S. R., Marsh, A. and Matheson, J. (1987) Explaining smokers' decisions to stop: Test of an expectancy-value approach. *Social Behaviour*, **2**, 35–49.

Velicer, W., Prochaska, J. O., Bellis, J. M. *et al.* (1993) An expert system intervention for smoking cessation. *Addictive Behaviors*, **18**, 269–90.

13

Group therapy and the addictions

WOJCIECH FALKOWSKI

Introduction

From the very early stages of childhood man is involved with and dependent on other people, and these experiences play a vital part in the development of personality. These years provide the foundations for later adaptive and maladaptive behaviour, and this early experience gives rise to development of what Berne (1975) called 'scripts', a term borrowed from theatrical terminology. He considered that the individual's life follows a certain pattern which is determined in childhood under the powerful influence of parental figures, as a result of which a person may behave as if he or she were an actor. As Shakespeare wrote:

All the world's a stage
And all the men and women merely players:
They have their exits and their entrances;
And one man in his time plays many parts

Shakespeare: As You Like It, II, vii, 139

Many interactions in group therapy are enactments of early childhood experiences and can readily be explored in the group setting. The aim of group psychotherapy is to provide a fuller and more accurate understanding of the self, and of the effect that an individual has on others in the group, and to evaluate the effect of others on the individual. Patients learn about themselves from the group leader and from other members of the group. They can discover how their behaviour and attitudes are often self-defeating and destructive, causing them to be misunderstood by others and causing others to misunderstand them. A cohesive, supportive, group can serve as a powerful encouragement in maintaining the patient's abstinence from drugs and alcohol.

Historical development of groups

Joseph Pratt (1908), an American physician, is often credited with being the father of group therapy. He started weekly 'classes' for the treatment of patients who had been rejected by sanatoria for the treatment of tuberculosis. The classes comprised 15 to 20 patients at a time and provided an opportunity for patients to learn more about their illness and to discuss and share their feelings with fellow patients. As a result of this supportive environment patients experienced an improvement in both morale and physical health.

Freud (1955) extended psychoanalytic insights into sociology and anthropology by studying crowd behaviour and the relationships of groups to their leaders. Despite these group studies he confined his attention to the examination of individual therapy. Similarly, Jung developed a distinct prejudice against the use of the group setting in his clinical work. This was possibly as a result of the orientation of his main thesis: that the personality is unique and therefore individual analysis is the crucial basis of such an approach to treatment. It is interesting, however, to note that a contemporary of Jung and Freud, Alfred Adler (Mosak and Dreikurs, 1973), considered that social factors, being both the cause and treatment of mental disorder, should form the basis of group treatment in child guidance and the treatment of alcoholics.

During and after the Second World War, it became apparent that a large patient population amongst the military could be efficiently treated in groups, and this gave impetus to the development of this form of therapy. In Britain the two prominent innovators were Bion (1961) and Foulkes (1946, 1964). Bion placed the emphasis on the interaction between the group and the leader. The leader adopts a passive, relatively opaque stance and interprets the group response towards the leader. Although of theoretical interest, this form of therapy is of limited value in running a group for drug addicts or alcoholics. Foulkes, who was also influenced by classical psychoanalysis, whilst not denying the importance of the analysis of interaction between the whole group and the therapist, drew attention to the importance of transference phenomena as arising between the individual members of the group towards the therapist and towards each other. He maintained that the feature that distinguishes group analysis from individual analysis is that transference patterns are more horizontal than vertical. In a group setting, the patient may respond transferentially to the therapist, to one or more patients, and even to the group as a whole. The analysis of such variety of transference phenomena has led to the description of unconscious forces operating within the group and the individual, and hopefully to psychotherapeutic insight.

In the United States, Kurt Lewin (1951) was greatly influenced by scientific theories in the field of physics and subsequently developed the theory of the individual being inescapably surrounded by social forces. This he called field theory. Over the years this has led to the development of various psychotherapeutic approaches such as sensitivity groups, focused on self-awareness and personal growth. Such ideas have also contributed to humanistic psychology.

Although the study of various approaches to group therapy is fascinating, for a therapist intending to learn how to lead a group this is best achieved through regular clinical supervision. Such novitiates might well at first confine themselves to a reading of an excellent textbook by Yalom (1975).

Advantages of group psychotherapy in treatment of alcohol and drug abusers

Group psychotherapy for alcoholics and drug addicts has been widely used (Madden and Kenyon, 1975; Blume, 1989; Wallace, 1989; Sandahl and Rosenberg, 1990; Lovet and Lovet, 1991; Mantano and Yalom, 1991; Vannicelli, 1991; Flores and Mahon, 1993; Kemker *et al.*, 1993). It has several advantages over individual psychotherapy, although both forms of therapy have a distinct place. Bowers and al-Redha (1990) have shown that the treatment of alcohol, drug, and marital problems can be carried out more effectively in a group than on an individual basis. Group therapy promotes the development of interpersonal relationships and mutual support among the patients; this can be especially helpful as many of them decide to sever contact with their former drinking and drug addict companions. Forging such new relationships raises patients' self-esteem, and enhances their motivation and expectation of successful therapy as they meet patients who are functioning well without drugs or alcohol, and this will be discussed again later in more detail. Since many of these patients have had complex and difficult previous personal relationships, they tend to project strong feelings from the past towards the therapist ('transference'). Such transference phenomena in these patients are easier to deal with within the group than in individual therapy. In the group, dependence upon therapist is less pronounced than in individual therapy, and tends to be diffused among other members. The setting allows the therapist and members of the group to observe directly and interpret each other's behaviour. It allows patients to examine their interpersonal relationships and social skills. Since denial is a frequent defence mechanism used by drug addicts and alcoholics (Amodeo, 1990), confrontation of such denial can be more effective in a setting where there may be not only a therapist to intervene, but also useful peer interaction. Furthermore, there is greater support and encouragement for adaptive attitudes and positive behavioural changes than in an individual situation. The economic advantages of group psychotherapy are readily apparent.

Selection and preparation of patients for group therapy

Each referred patient should be individually interviewed by the therapist before entering the group. The patient may not be suitable, or may be more appropriate for a different group. Some patients may still be suffering from acute drug or alcohol withdrawal. Others may have psychotic symptoms, whether due to substance abuse or a result of underlying illness. Such patients should be excluded or considered only after their recovery from these conditions. Alcoholics or drug addicts who share additional problems such as having experiencd incest (Winick *et al.*, 1992) or who have suffered from psychotic illness (Nigam *et al.*, 1992), may benefit from specific groups. Similarly, many patients may derive benefit from family therapy groups (O'Farrell, 1989; McCrady, 1989; Reichelt and Christensen, 1990; Romijn *et al.*, 1990, 1992), or group therapy with couples (Bowers and al-Redha 1990; Salinas *et al.*, 1991).

There is an advantage in group membership being heterogenous; for example, in relation to age and sex. This provides the opportunity for wider dynamic exploration and group interaction. A very small group, for example of four patients, is not to be recommended. On the other hand, in a group of more than 12 patients, there is a risk that each member may not have the opportunity to be sufficiently involved in the group, and excessively large groups may lack group identity and cohesion. There is some evidence (Yalom *et al.*, 1967; Strupp and Bloxom, 1973; Bednar and Battersby, 1976) that introductory sessions can be of benefit before actual therapy starts. It is helpful if alcoholics or drug addicts have such introductory sessions from a professional other than their own group leader. At these sessions they can learn about the physical, social, and psychological effects of substance abuse. This would not only enable patients to acquire the requisite factual knowledge but would also allow them subsequently, in group therapy, to deal with

personal issues rather than, for instance, having prolonged discussions
about the effects of drugs or alcohol.

An extension of these didactic sessions can be followed by further
introductory sessions aiming at providing patients with a simple and
easy to understand psychological framework that will assist them in
comprehending the nature of common patterns of feelings and behaviour.
If patients are to be prepared for the group by way of such talks, this may
be most usefully carried out in the form of six introductory talks, including a brief exposition on theories of personality. This often helps patients
to understand their psychopathological state, trace its origin from past
life experiences, and understand the effect that they exert by their behaviour on other people and reciprocal influences. The theoretical framework that is most accessible to patients appears to be transactional
analysis (Falkowski, 1988; Falkowski and Falkowski, 1990; Falkowski
and Haslam, 1992). Kapur and Miller (1987) compared therapeutic factors in transactional analysis and psychodynamic group psychotherapy,
and found that there was more emphasis on individual problems within
the group in transactional analysis as compared to psychodynamic psychotherapy. Regrettably, group therapy for some alcoholics and drug
addicts is not always beneficial. There is little research into the selection
criteria for patients who are likely to respond to group therapy.

Rules and expectations

Careful consideration should be given to whether or not the patient
should be allowed to attend another form of therapy. For instance, a
patient simultaneously in individual therapy may avoid confronting
important issues by reporting that he is dealing with these issues in individual therapy and vice versa. Different therapist orientations and styles
may lead to confusion, for patient and therapist alike.

It is important that the group therapist should not reveal the intended
specific composition of the group as this may prevent spontaneous and
often irrational reactions to occur, which could then be usefully explored.
Patients should be told about the purpose of the group and asked to
agree to conform to certain rules, such as complete abstinence from
drugs (other than medically prescribed), to inform personally if unable
to attend the group, to attend punctually and to observe complete confidentiality. Since many patients are frightened of being in group therapy,
especially in early stages, and find themselves rather lost, it is good policy
to obtain initial agreement from patients that they will attend at least four

sessions before deciding finally whether to discontinue attending the group. Similarly, it is useful if the patient who feels that he or she has completed treatment will announce his or her intention of leaving the group four sessions before doing so. It often happens that someone announces the intention to leave the group, but later discovers that the real reason for talking about quitting was the reluctance to deal with important, difficult and painful issues. These four sessions frequently give the patient opportunity to evaluate his or her real motivation, and often therapy is then continued. However, a patient who has achieved his or her desired goal in therapy, made satisfactory adjustment to life and is appropriately ready to leave the group will have the opportunity gradually to detach from the group, and the group members will be able to go through the separation process. This is also an opportunity to affirm the patient's achievement, and is encouraging for the group.

Clear rules should be established governing patients who come to the group drinking or taking drugs, and patients should be aware of these at the outset. If it becomes necessary to enforce these rules, this should be done firmly but with tact and compassion. The patient who comes to the group drunk or takes drugs should be asked to leave and come to the next group only if completely abstinent. Sometimes a relapse is caused by an obvious precipitant such as an unexpected death in the family and the patient may subsequently remain completely abstinent. A relapse may present the opportunity to examine in what way the patient is unable to cope with stress and this may help him to develop adaptive ways of coping with life without substance abuse. Further, those who drink or take drugs between the groups should agree to desist from doing so or be excluded from the group. If a patient continues relapsing he should be excluded for a period of time. A disruptive patient who frequently relapses should be excluded from the group permanently.

It is helpful for the group therapist to have a co-therapist. It allows the therapist after each session to discuss process and content, offers therapists mutual support, and if one is unable to attend the other can supply continuity. Group leaders often have little opportunity for proper training or are trained to conduct only general groups.

An open group is one where new members can enter at any time, as opposed to a 'closed' group where all members start and terminate together with no new members along the route. The group sessions should take place in the same room, at the same day of the week, and the same time. They should start and end punctually. The best duration is usually one and a half hours, but can be longer, subject to previous mutual agreement. There should be no table in the middle of the room, as this impairs non-verbal communication.

Early stages of group treatment

Patients invariably come into a group with a great deal of anxiety, fear, and ambivalence. Some patients may doubt the relevance of this method of treatment to their problems; some are resentful, angry, and covertly hostile at having been coerced into treatment by employers or pressure from relatives. Failure to recognise these undercurrents and to deal with them effectively and tactfully, may result in the formation of undue resistance, slow down therapeutic progress, or even cause the patient to stop attending. Some patients may invest the therapist with magical powers to solve their problems, and expect him or her to have ready answers to all dilemmas. Early successful resolution of these difficulties will contribute to the group cohesion that is essential for successful therapy.

Patients who suffer trauma, deprivation, and arrest of healthy emotional development at an earlier age will have particular difficulties in relating to the group and therapist, and will require tolerance and support. The most important and frequently encountered defence mechanism in the initial stages of therapeutic work is denial of the drink or drug problem (Amodeo, 1990). Some patients may have no trust in the therapist or the group, and believe that they cannot cope with life stresses without drugs or alcohol. One can frequently hear such statements as 'I can stop drinking any time I wish, I do not have a drink problem', or 'Drink is an essential part of successful business transactions'. Other variants of defence are 'If I discover why I am drinking, I will stop', 'I can't stop drinking because my life has been ruined, my business collapsed and my wife left me', or 'What is the point of trying, no one here seems to understand me or tries to help'.

Such statements are supported by psychological defence mechanisms that protect the patient against dealing with deep problems that would induce intolerable anxiety and emotional pain. If these issues are not successfully dealt with the patient becomes a victim of his or her defences. Considerable therapeutic skill is essential in dealing with these matters. Patients may need to be confronted, and such confrontations have to be well timed, and should be specific and based on undisputed objective evidence. For instance, the author asked a patient who maintained that he had no drinking problem to convince his liver of this fact (liver functions were distinctly abnormal). This created a certain amount of benevolent amusement in the group, and the patient immediately changed his attitude in the desired direction.

Confrontation must be delivered with care and genuine concern, as otherwise the patient will perceive it as an attack and become more entrenched in a position. The therapist must guard against expressing attitudes that are judgemental, punitive, moralistic, or superior. The patient should not feel humiliated, and there should be no winners or losers. Ideally, confrontation should only be given to the patient when he or she is not too distressed, and only when there is sufficient cohesion and support in the group and tension is not too high. When a patient gains insight, encouragement, positive feedback ('strokes' in terms of transactional analysis), protection, concern and attention may all be needed.

Generally, insight therapy should be resisted while the patient is abusing alcohol or drugs, no matter how interesting the underlying psychopathological reasons for drinking or drug-taking may appear to the therapist. Continuing abuse of these substances will inhibit therapeutic progress, and may seriously damage or even kill the patient before the cause of addictive behaviour is established. On the other hand, discovery of the unconscious reasons for drinking or drug abuse, although important, does not necessarily guarantee recovery.

Abstinence from drugs and alcohol may initially be very stressful, but will lead to the amelioration of physical and mental discomfort and improvement of unsocial functioning. Early sobriety is, though, frequently associated with having to face difficulties and responsibilities that the patient was able to ignore while drinking or taking drugs. They may be faced with relentless guilt, which can in turn lead to recurrent relapse. Some patients will adopt a 'medical model', and see themselves as suffering from an illness. While such an attitude is helpful in reducing the stigma of being a drug addict or alcoholic, it may lead the patient to adopt a passive role – 'It's an illness, I can't help it'.

Group therapists, particularly if inexperienced and especially at the early stages of the group, are likely to encounter a level of anxiety that is based on the need to maintain a good self-image and the approval of their supervisors, and their wish to gain control of the group. They may be afraid of the group disintegrating, of undue resistances or hostility developing, or of unmanageable multiple transferences. Therapists may develop strong positive and negative transferences towards some members of the group, which are handicapping. Regular supervision is therefore strongly indicated. Many group therapists who work with substance problems have no formal training in group psychotherapy and are them-selves 'in recovery'. While some patients will be greatly encouraged by this kind of group leadership, through the process of 'identification', such therapists are specially likely to need support and supervision.

Later stages of group psychotherapy

In the early stages of group development patients are uncertain of their position, and tend to be over-adaptive, conforming, and over-sensitive towards the leader's comments and interpretations, which they are liable to understand as criticism of themselves. Patients may develop a variety of behaviours to escape dealing with important aspects of psychopathol-ogy by, for instance, coming late to the group. Other patients volunteer to present minor issues, sometimes even to the extent of inventing a problem that they do not have. As the group progresses, resentments, hostilities towards some members and attraction to other group members may develop. These feelings and interactions can temporarily slow down the therapeutic progress. Hostile comments towards other group members may really be a covert attack on the therapist.

In course of time, patients acquire ability to express fear, dependency, anxiety, anger, jealousy and other distressing feelings. They relate painful past experiences and will identify with each others' problems and diffi-culties. They learn to confront each other in a caring, constructive way. The therapist is likely to be viewed as expert in therapy, but nevertheless as someone with human fallibility.

Therapeutic factors in group therapy

Detailed knowledge of the various theories of group therapy does not appear to be in practice helpful when conducting a group for alcoholics or drug addicts. Corsini and Rosenberg (1955) identified those compo-nents that are commonly viewed by all schools of group therapy as therapeutic (although there is no proven external evidence that they are in fact therapeutic and they were derived from clinical observation rather than having a research basis. Separation between them is somewhat arbi-trary. Nevertheless, they offer a useful framework for understanding the interactions that go on within any group). These factors were further elaborated by Yalom (1975) and subsequently modified by Bloch *et al.* (1979) and Bloch and Crouch (1985). They can be summarised as acceptance (patient feels accepted by the group, an integral part of cohesiveness); altruism (capacity to help other group members); universality (feeling 'we are all in the same boat'); installation of hope (to successful outcome); vicarious learning (by observation of group member's interaction); guidance (information or advice received within the group); self-understanding; learning from interpersonal actions (acquisition of more adaptive behaviour within the group); self-disclosure; and catharsis.

Some of these factors are particularly pertinent to group treatment for substance misuse. This universality is important and it enables such patients to share emotions and problems in an open and honest way, and leads to altruism and other therapeutic developments. Members of a cohesive group with strong group identity tend to have good outcome (Yalom and Rand, 1966; Maxmen and Hanover, 1973; Yalom, 1975; Butler and Fuhriman, 1983; Marcovitz and Smith, 1983; Bloch and Crouch, 1985). Varieties of self-help groups have been developing in the last 30 years, and the contribution of AA and Narcotic Anonymous cannot be overlooked. Universality and other factors important in these groups are discussed in detail by Ephraim (1988).

Closely related to universality is the concept of identification. There is some suggestion that identification with the therapist is a salient component in group therapy. Kissen (1974) speculated that the degree of identification with the therapist by patients is influenced by such therapist characteristics as style of expression, social status, and perceived competence. Jeske (1993) suggested that clinical improvement was related to identification during group therapy, and that the therapist should consciously encourage an identification process in the group. Identification is often associated with modelling. Modelling in group therapy consists of observation of another person's behaviour, remembering it, and subsequently behaving in a similar manner. It is, put simply, learning by an example. Thus a patient may discover how to become more assertive in a group, and less anxious of being open. A particular technique for declining an offer of an alcoholic drink in a social situation may be learnt. Modelling may result in productive or unproductive behaviour, and the relapse into drinking of one patient is not infrequently followed by relapse of one or two others. Modelling and identification are probably prominent factors in psychodrama. Psychodrama (Loughlin, 1992), Gestalt and other 'Action Therapies' (Falkowski, 1991), can be useful as major approaches, or various action therapy methods can be used during conventional therapy sessions, especially when the group reaches 'plateau' due to resistance (Falkowski, 1988; Crawford, 1989, Getter *et al.*, 1991).

As a patient's self-esteem and confidence increases, he or she will often extend help to other members of the group and thus display altruism. This can be of value in that when a patient offers support or gives useful suggestions he or she will feel needed and helpful, and self-esteem is likely to increase. Altruism also serves indirectly in promoting sensitivity and lessening self-absorption (Bloch and Crouch, 1985; Ephraim, 1988). 'Installation of hope' (Yalom, 1975), the expectation that the patient has a chance to succeed in therapy, can be a powerful therapeutic factor in the group and particularly in an open group. Vicarious learning can apply to achievement and maintenance of abstinence, and can also help members of the group to make better adjustments in everyday life, improve relationhips wth a spouse, get on better at work, and so on.

It is rewarding to ask members of the group to review their progress at regular intervals. The therapist has to be aware of the envy and anger that this procedure may instigate in some members. Transactional analysis may be helpful in setting 'contracts' and reviewing and rewarding progress (Stewart and Jones, 1989).

Despite very common use of group therapy in alcoholism and drug addiction there are few controlled studies in this area and even these have serious methodological limitations (Brandsma and Patterson, 1985). We need to review our own progress.

References

Amodeo, M. (1990) Treating the late-life alcoholic: guidelines for working through denial and integrating individual, family, and group approaches. *Journal of Geriatric Psychiatry*, **23**, 91–105.

Bednar, R. L. and Battersby, C. P. (1976) The effects of specific cognitive structure on early group development. *Journal of Applied Behavioural Science*, **12**, 513–22.

Berne, E. (1975) *Transactional Analysis in Psychotherapy*. London: Souvenir Press. (Originally published in 1961 by Balantine Books, New York.)

Bion, W. (1961) *Experiences in Groups*. London: Tavistock.

Bloch, S. and Crouch, E. (1985) *Therapeutic Factors in Group Psychotherapy*, pp. 99–123. Oxford: Oxford University Press.

Bloch, S., Reibstein, J., Crouch, E., Holroyd, P. and Theman, J. (1979) A method of the study of therapeutic factors in group psychotherapy. *British Journal of Psychiatry*, **134**, 257–63.

Blume, S. B. (1989) Treatment for addictions in a psychiatric setting. *British Journal of Addiction*, **84**, 727–9.

Bowers, T. G. and al-Redha, M. R. (1990) A comparison of outcome with group/marital and standard/individual therapies with alcoholics. *Journal of Studies on Alcohol*, **51**, 301–9.

Brandsma, J. M. and Patterson, E. M. (1985) The outcome of group psychotherapy for alcoholics: an empirical review. *American Journal of Drug and Alcohol Abuse*, **11**, 151–62.

Butler, T. and Fuhriman, A. (1983) Level of functioning and length of time in treatment variables influencing patients' therapeutic experience in group psychotherapy. *International Journal of Group Psychotherapy*, **33**, 489–504.

Corsini, R. and Rosenberg, B. (1955) Mechanisms of group psychotherapy: process and dynamics. *Journal of Abnormal and Social Psychology*, **51**, 406–11.

Crawford, R. J. (1989) Follow up of alcohol and other drug dependents treated with psychodrama. *New Zealand Medical Journal*, **102**, 199–200.

Ephraim, N. W. (1988) In: Aveline, M. and Dryden, W. (eds.) *Self-help Groups in Group Therapy in Britain*, pp. 233–54. Milton Keynes, Philadelphia: Open University Press.

Falkowski, W. (1988) Action Therapy. *Postgraduate Doctor*, **10**, 17–22.

Falkowski, W. (1991) A brief outline of transactional psychotherapy. *Postgraduate Doctor*, **12**, 28–34.

Falkowski, W. and Falkowski, J. (1990) Alcohol: Our favourite poison. *Maternal and Child Health*, **15**, 130–7.

Falkowski, W. and Haslam, M. T. (1992) Function of a community centre in treatment of alcoholism. *Journal of the Hong Kong College of Psychiatrists*, **2**, 33–6.

Flores, P. J. and Mahon, L. (1993) The treatment of addiction in group psychotherapy. *International Journal of Group Psychotherapy*, **43**, 143–56.

Foulkes, S. H. (1946) Group analysis in a military neurosis centre. *Lancet*, **1**, 303–6.

Foulkes, S. H. (1964) *Therapeutic Group Analysis*. London: Allen Unwin.

Freud, S. (1955) *Group Psychology and the Analysis of the Ego*. London: Hogarth Press.

Getter, H., Kadden, R. M. and Cooney, N. L. (1991) Measuring treatment process in coping skills and interactional group therapies for alcoholism. *International Journal of Group Psychotherapy*, **42**, 419–30.

Jeske, O. (1993) Identification and therapeutic effectiveness in group therapy. *Journal of Counselling Psychology*, **20**, 528–30.

Kapur, R. and Miller, K. (1987) A comparison between therapeutic factors in TA and psychodynamic therapy groups. *Transactional Analysis Journal*, **17**, 294–300.

Kemker, S. S., Kibel, H. D. and Mahler, J. C. (1993) On becoming oriented to impatient addiction treatment: inducing new patients and professionals to recovery movement. *International Journal of Group Psychotherapy*, **43**, 285–301.

Kissen, M. (1974) The concept of identification: an evaluation of its curent status and its significance for group psychotherapy. In: Rasenbaum, M. (ed.) *Group Psychotherapy from the South-West*, pp. 25–36. New York: Gordon and Breach.

Lewin, K. (1951) *Field Theory in Social Science*. New York: Harper.

Loughlin, N. (1992) A trial of the use of psychodrama with alcohol problems. *Nursing Practice*, **5**, 14–19.

Lovet, L. and Lovet, J. (1991) Group therapeutic factors on an alcohol in-patient unit. *British Journal of Psychiatry*, **159**, 365–70.

Madden, J. S. and Kenyon, W. H. (1975) Group counselling of alcoholics by a voluntary agency. *British Journal of Psychiatry*, **126**, 289–91.

Marcovitz, R. J. and Smith, J. E. (1983) Patients' perception of curative factors in short-term group psychotherapy. *International Journal of Group Psychotherapy*, **33**, 21–39.

Matano, R. A. and Yalom, I. D. (1991) Approaches to chemical dependency: chemical dependency and interactive group therapy – a synthesis. *International Journal of Group Psychotherapy*, **41**, 269–93.

Maxmen, J. S. and Hanover, J. D. (1973) Group psychotherapy as viewed by hospitalized patients. *Archives of General Psychiatry*, **28**, 404–8.

McCrady, B. S. (1989) Outcome of family-involved alcoholism treatment. *Recent Developments in Alcoholism*, **7**, 165–82.

Mosak, H. H. and Dreikurs, R. (1973) Adlerian psychotherapy. In: Corsini, R. (ed.) *Psychotherapies*, pp. 44–94. Itasca: Peacock.

Nigam, R., Schottenfeld, R. and Kosten, T. R. (1992) Treatment of dual diagnosis patients: a relapse prevention group approach. *Journal of Substance Abuse Treatment*, **9**, 305–9.

O'Farrell, T. J. (1989) Marital and family therapy in alcoholism treatment. *Journal of Substance Abuse Treatment*, **8**, 23–9.

Pratt, J. H. (1908) *The Tuberculosis Class. An Experiment in Home Treatment in Group Therapy and Group Function* (ed. Rosenbaum, M. and Berger, M.). New York: Basic Books, 1975.

Reichelt, S. and Christensen, B. (1990) Reflections during a study on family therapy with drug addicts. *Family Process*, **29**, 273–87.

Romijn, C. M., Platt, J. J. and Schippers, G. M. (1990) Family therapy for Dutch drug abusers: replication of an American study. *International Journal of Addictions*, **25**, 1127–49.

Romijn, C. M., Platt, J. J., Schippers, G. M. and Schaap, C. P. (1992) Family therapy for Dutch drug users: the relationship between family functioning and success. *International Journal of Addictions*, **27**, 1–14.

Salinas, R. C., O'Farrell, T. J., Jones, W. C. and Cutter, H. S. 1991) Services for families of Alcoholics: a national survey of Veteran Affairs treatment programs. *Journal of Studies on Alcohol*, **52**, 541–6.

Sandahl, C. and Rosenberg, S. (1990) Brief group psychotherapy in relapse prevention for alcohol dependent patients. *International Journal of Group Psychotherapy*, **40**, 453–76.

Stewart, I. and Jones, V. (1989) *TA Today. A New Introduction to Transactional Analysis.* Nottingham and Chapel Hill: Lifespace Publishing.

Strupp, H. H. and Bloxom, A. L. (1973) Preparing lower-class patients for group psychotherapy. *Journal of Consulting and Clinical Psychology*, **41**, 373–84.

Vannicelli, M. (1991) Dilemma of countertransference considerations in group psychotherapy with adult children of alcoholics. *International Journal of Group Psychotherapy*, **41**, 295–312.

Wallace, B. C. (1989) Relapse prevention in psycho-educational groups for compulsive crack cocaine smokers. *Journal of Substance Abuse Treatment*, **6**, 229–39.

Winick, C., Levine, A. and Stone, W. A. (1992) An incest survivors' therapy group. *Journal of Substance Abuse Treatment*, **9**, 311–8.

Yalom, I. D. (1975) *The Theory and Practice of Group Psychotherapy.* New York: Basic Books.

Yalom, I. D., Houts, P. S. and Newell, G. (1967) Preparation of patients for group therapy: a controlled study. *Archives of General Psychiatry*, **17**, 416–27.

Yalom, I. D. and Rand, K. (1966) Compatability and cohesiveness in therapy groups. *Archives of General Psychiatry*, **15**, 267–75.

14

Alcoholics Anonymous as mirror held up to nature

GRIFFITH EDWARDS

Introduction

A drinking problem is in its essence a feeling and behaviour towards oneself and other people, which is embedded in the drinker's personal history and situated within the nexus of a total, complex, personal present. Recovery, when it begins to arrive, will be based on the individual's own sense of possibilities for change and movement within that subjective and objective, constraining and enabling, historically and contemporarily determined reality. Recovery can be assisted by the therapist, but cannot be dictated by any professional outsider. The role of therapy is best considered as that of supporting a natural potential for recovery by perhaps a timely nudge, lending some hope, explaining techniques for self-management, or given a warning of blind alleys.

That perspective was articulated by Orford and Edwards (1977) in the following terms:

The influences, whether non-specific or specific, which go under the heading of 'treatment' do not impinge on an individual who is isolated from all other influences. On the contrary, treatment or advice should be seen as elements added to, and inter-reacting with, a continuously evolving field of what might be termed *natural influences*. . . Therapy may not in itself be a particularly powerful force, but if we understand the natural balance of forces, the balance may be favourably tipped.

That is not a denigratory, nihilistic view of treatment, but it differs radically from the concept of any single favoured intervention as sovereign and specific remedy, a master stroke to be prescribed for the patient who is the passive recipient of a powerful medicine.

The argument that sees the understanding of 'natural healing processes' as the best foundation for treatment of drinking problems has been further developed by Vaillant (1980), with empirical support from his own longitudinal research (Vaillant, 1983). Of particular relevance to the concerns of the present chapter is the suggestion made by Vaillant (1980) that AA may contain within it important elements of what studies of the drinker's career reveal as being the possible levers or processes that effect change in drinking and life course over the longer term:

The success of Alcoholics Anonymous and its facsimiles . . . is probably due to the fact that it conforms so well to the natural healing principles.

Alcoholics Anonymous, Vaillant seems to be suggesting, is a mirror to be held up to nature, and in which we may see reflected the natural processes of healing. AA was not created by doctors or psychologists, or within the views of any profession as to what was to be deemed to be good for the patients, and it was not designed with regard to any stated theory. Rather, AA happened and evolved in response to a chance meeting in 1935 between two drunken Americans (Alcoholics Anonymous, 1976), has evolved into a fellowship with an estimated two million members worldwide, and with a capacity to adapt to a diversity of cultures (Mäkelä, 1991). The question of 'whether AA works' in terms of its ability positively to influence individual drinking outcome is one to which we will return later, but what meanwhile stands out as a fact in its own right is that people have over the years and in their millions, voted with their feet.

The framework for this chapter will be as follows. An account will first be provided of AA's ideology and mode of operation. In the next section an attempt will be made to identify the elements within the overall AA process that support change. Finally, attention will be focused on the question of what professionals can, in sum, learn from AA.

Within the space available, the discussion of the relevant research literature must inevitably be selective, and note should therefore be taken of a recent and comprehensive review volume (McCrady and Miller, 1993). There is also an extensive, older literature on AA that is still of interest (Bales, 1944; Tiebout, 1944; Bacon, 1957; Cooper and Maule, 1962). The focus will be on Alcoholics Anonymous, rather than on Alanon, Alateen, Narcotics Anonymous, or those numerous other organisations that have built on, or borrowed from, AA, and which today contribute to the variety and intensity of 'Twelve Steps' or self-help consciousness (Robinson and Henry, 1977; Room, 1993). Neither will we deal with 'The Minnesota Model' (Cook, 1988*a,b*).

AA: ideology, organisational basis, and mode of operation

Authoritative statements on AA's beliefs and functioning are to be found in several publications emanating from the fellowship itself (Alcoholics Anonymous, 1952, 1976, 1990). Descriptions have also been given by outside commentators (for instance, Robinson, 1979; Edwards, 1987).

The Twelve Steps

The fundamentals of AA's belief system are authoritatively stated in the Twelve Steps, which are reproduced below in full.

1. We admitted we were powerless over alcohol – that our lives had become unmanageable.
2. Came to believe that a Power greater than ourselves could restore us to sanity.
3. Made a decision to turn our will and our lives over to the care of God *as we understand Him*.
4. Made a searching and fearless inventory of ourselves.
5. Admitted to God, to ourselves and to another human being the exact nature of our wrongs.
6. Were entirely ready to have God remove all these defects of character.
7. Humbly asked Him to remove our shortcomings.
8. Made a list of all persons we had harmed, and became willing to make amends to them all.
9. Made direct amends to such people wherever possible, except when to do so would injure them or others.
10. Continued to take personal inventory and when we were wrong, promply admitted it.
11. Sought through prayer and meditation to improve our conscious contact with God *as we understand Him*, praying only for knowledge of His will for us and the power to carry that out.
12. Having a spiritual awakening as the result of these steps, we tried to carry this message to alcoholics and to practice these principles in all our affairs.

Different AA members may find varied meanings in this formulation, but what it undoubtedly comprises is both a flexible belief system and an action programme. Some notes of exegesis may be helpful.

Step 1 is an admission of powerlessness, of 'having reached rock bottom', or of 'surrender' (Tiebout, 1953), and is often seen as the necessary precondition to entering the AA recovery programme. 'Rock bottom' does not necessarily mean destitution, and the thinking here is not to be misinterpreted as implying that the drinker can only be helped after experiencing the ultimates of personal loss. The needed turning point may be simply a sense of not being able to go on this way, of enough being enough, of 'being sick and tired of being sick and tired'.

Step 2 invites belief in a higher Power, while **Step 3** refers to 'God as we understand him'. These and the further references to God that occur in Steps 5, 6, 7 and 11 might on first reading be interpreted as suggesting that AA is a religious sect still tied rather closely to its Oxford Group origins. In practice the individual member is likely to put a personal meaning on the concept of a higher power which can range all the way from an orthodox religious interpretation to that power conceived in lay terms as being within the conjoined strength of the Fellowship itself. Atheism is no bar to membership. We will return later (p. 235) to a further consideration of the spiritual dimension within AA.

Step 4 involves making 'a moral inventory of ourselves'. This is likely to be interpreted as demanding a tangible exercise in self-appraisal rather than as its being satisfied by an abstract statement of intent.

Step 5 the admission to some other person of the 'exact nature' of the individual's wrong doing, is again a step to be given practical meaning.

Step 6 refers to 'defects of character', while **Step 7** asks for their removal. The programme thus confronts the AA member with the need to achieve deep inner change rather than tackle the drinking behaviour in isolation.

Step 8 and **Step 9** deal with the need to make good any harm done to others – the act of reparation.

Step 10 refers again to the need for personal inventory, thus emphasising that the commitment to change cannot be satisfied by any one-off act.

Step 11 which encourages 'prayer and meditation' is overtly theistic, but is probably interpreted by many AA members as indicating the need for contemplation and quiet time, rather than commitment to any orthodoxy.

Step 12, the final step in the programme, indicates that the person who has achieved his or her own 'spiritual awakening' should be willing to give back to others. The phrase 'twelfth stepping' is used to describe the involvement of the established AA member in helping the newcomer. Formal responsibility will be taken for 'sponsoring' someone who has recently joined (see p. 228), but such involvement is limited to helping people who want to be helped. Prosletysing, searching the highways and byways for new recruits, or 'pulling drunks down lamp-posts', is no part of the job. Sponsorship is not something to be attempted prematurely and older members will warn against trying too hard, excesses of enthusiasm, or putting one's own sobriety at risk.

The Twelve Steps thus define a pathway. One step will be attempted before the next in sequence, thought will be required and advice given as to how swiftly progression is to be made, and progress may be at a very varied personal pace along this path. Some members may use the steps as providing structured guidance for personal development over a lifetime, while others may engage in and enjoy AA, but with a much less formal commitment to working the Twelve Steps. Available for everyone either as master plan or occasional reference is, however, a signposted, stepwise programme for recovery.

AA beliefs as to the nature of the drinking problem

The Twelve Steps are remarkable for their scant mention of drink. 'Alcohol' gets a mention in Step 1 and 'alcoholics' in Step 12, but between these two points there is nothing directly to suggest that AA is a self-help group for people who are worried about their drinking. One can only assume that this drafting reflects the early Oxford Group influence, with a consequent general emphasis on repentance, confession, redemption, making good, and religious conversion.

Despite the seeming relative neglect of drinking in this founding delineation of the AA programme, the fellowship has in practice and on the basis of oral tradition, an explicit formulation of the nature of the drinking problem as 'alcoholism', with alcoholism a disease. The disease is physical, psychological, and spiritual. Once an alcoholic always an alcoholic. The disease can be arrested by sobriety, but is never cured. Metaphorically, alcoholism is an allergy to alcohol. Through no fault of their own, 'sick alcoholics' will never be able to handle alcohol again safely. The AA member is 'in recovery', but never recovered. The requirement is for life-time vigilance, and 'the first drink is the one you can't afford'.

Thus to a stepwise programme of recovery is added a matching formulation on the nature of the disorder. Both the recovery programme and the identification of alcoholism as disease can be construed as simple and readily intelligible formulations designed to relieve the confusion of the person walking through the door to his or her first AA meeting. The deeper subtleties residing in the Twelve Steps or in the concept of a 'disease' that affects body, mind and soul, should not however be underestimated. These complexities will be explored only long after that first meeting, but the AA ideology offers plentiful invitations to debate. For its members, however, the AA tradition seems, happily, more to invite a searching after personal understanding than engagements in doctrinal dispute. *Odium theologicam*, the hatred that characterises theological dissensions, is not an AA disease.

The AA meeting

The central everyday event in the AA calendar is the AA meeting, which will be organised with fixed regularity of time and place by each local AA group (Thursdays, say, at 7.30 p.m., at the St Barnabas Community Centre). The group has its own elected treasurer and secretary. A chairman will be chosen for the occasion, and a speaker introduced who is an AA member from this or a neighbouring group. There will probably be about 10–20 people present, but the meeting can be larger or smaller. There are no subscriptions, nor is there any formal mechanism for enrolment. Meetings may be 'closed' and thus restricted to people who define themselves as alcoholics, or 'open' and welcoming to all comers. Anonymity is the rule, and only first names are used.

Ceremony is at a minimum. A speaker will introduce himself or herself, with the phrase 'My name is . . . and I'm an alcoholic', a formula that invites identification and rejects stigma.

Soundings suggest that there are keen judgements on the difference between an empathetic and a tedious speaker, but good manners will always rule the day and no one is interrupted. The speaker who is most appreciated is likely to be the one who talks positively about recovery rather than dwelling too much on the pains of the drinking past, and who is able to convey a sense of hope. An element of homespun wisdom, a few old saws, and some flashes of humour also make for a good mix. There is, however, no one structure for this kind of presentation. The aim is not rhetoric or the winning of applause, but 'sharing'. An AA story is an art form that allows many variations, but is never a sermon.

There are no formal rules for the floor discussion that follows the opening speaker's contribution, but tradition seems to propose that each statement stands in its own right. The meeting is a place for saying something about oneself, rather than for sharp debate, criticism or attack, or the pursuit of intellectual abstractions. If advice is given directly to someone else, it is likely to be in response to a tangible request for help, and it will be low key, a matter of 'it's only my opinion'. AA is never an Encounter Group. Older hands will be likely to return time and again during the course of a meeting to the need for a simple, workable personal strategy for staying sober. AA members will learn at an early stage that the task is to stay sober 'a day at a time' and not to make great promises, nor become too burdened by the future. The 'recovering alcoholic' should be aware of the dangers that can lie in self-deception and particularly in the habit of blaming other people, and will be reminded that the problem is 'not just your drinking but your stinking thinking'. If you are getting into an argument, walk away, 'count ten'. The danger of becoming over-confident, cocksure, or of letting down one's guard, will be repeatedly warned against. AA is often about saying the same thing again and again, with humour, with conviction, backed by personal experience, and with the practical applications made evident.

Although there are repeated themes, each meeting will be different. The meetings may be low-key, but the effect of the opening talk and the further contributions can, in sum, be powerful. Group cohesion is built and the overall belief system reinforced, skills for survival are learnt, things are said that can be taken away, and hope is given.

At the end of the meeting there is time for coffee or tea and for informal interchange. A new member need not have said anything, will not have been probed or questioned, but will have been made welcome.

AA experiences outside the meeting

Although the group meeting is a highly significant part of the AA experience, the totality of the AA experience can go much wider. Most pervasively, the individual who is truly involved with AA will be 'on the programme' and applying the AA message to daily living. There will be a parallel with the behaviour therapist's prescription of homework, with AA precepts tested out in their practical application rather than left at the intellectual level. There may be a reporting back at the next meeting of small but significant successes (a drink refused, a charged emotional situation not taken as excuse for drinking, someone else's point of view seen). An AA card may be carried in the pocket with the Twelve Steps listed and with the Serenity Prayer as talisman against the difficult moment:

God grant me the serenity
To accept the things I cannot change
The courage to change the things I can
And the wisdom to know the difference

Contact with other members that continues outside group meetings may be initiated at the first encounter with AA. This may be a matter of no more than a couple of telephone numbers for support, or a few people having a meal together on the way home. Later an arrangement may be set up for the new member whereby an experienced AA member acts as sponsor and takes more or less formal responsibility for Twelve Stepping the newcomer.

The fullest account of the broad and diverse range of activities and social involvements that can evolve from AA membership has been given by Robinson (1979), on the basis of a survey of London AA attenders. He described the elements that can make up 'AA as a way of life'. New friendships are made that may often lead to shared leisure activities, and visits to each other's houses, with family involvement. Conferences and conventions will be attended. Time may be given to running AA's switchboard, and in time many members will share in office-holding responsibilities at group level. AA literature will be read, and study groups may be attended. Talks on AA may be given to professional groups and outside audiences.

Thus, although AA meetings have been described as 'a speech event', a full understanding of AA's ability to attract, hold, and re-socialise the individual in sobriety, requires a much wider awareness of activities and processes than those limited to the group meeting.

Organisation, but the minimum of bureaucracy

The basics of the AA organisational framework are contained in the Twelve Traditions (Alcoholics Anonymous, 1952):

1. Our common welfare should come first; personal recovery depends upon AA unity.
2. For our group purpose there is but one ultimate authority – a loving God as he may express Himself in our group conscience. Our leaders are but trusted servants; they do not govern.
3. The only requirement for AA membership is a desire to stop drinking.

4. Each group should be autonomous except in matters affecting other groups or AA as a whole.
5. Each group has but one primary purpose – to carry its message to the alcoholic who still suffers.
6. An AA group ought never endorse, finance or lend the AA name to any related facility or outside enterprise lest problems of money, property and prestige divert us from our primary purpose.
7. Every AA group ought to be fully self-supporting, declining outside contributions.
8. Alcoholics Anonymous should remain forever non-professional, but our service centers may employ special workers.
9. AA, as such, ought never be organized; but we may create service boards or committees directly responsible to those they serve.
10. Alcoholics Anonymous has no opinion on outside issues; hence the AA name ought never be drawn into public controversy.
11. Our public relations policy is based on attraction rather than promotion; we need always to maintain personal anonymity at the level of press, radio and films.
12. Anonymity is the spiritual foundation of our traditions, ever reminding us to place principles before personalities.

For present purposes it is unnecessary to analyse this statement item by item. It constitutes both a set of organisational precepts that offer guidance for good management, and warnings to avert any developments that could result either in schism or a too great involvement in worldly concerns. With the local group as the fundamental unit of organisation, co-ordination is effected through Intergroup meetings and then at national level by a General Services Board. The General Service Conference is an annual delegate meeting with decision-making responsibilities.

The overall administrative structure that supports AA's extensive local, national, and international operation is thus remarkable in several different ways. The Twelve Traditions fuse an element of mission statement with practical rules for business, and the organisational system derives from and supports AA's ethical and belief system. The organisational framework is constructed around flexible guidelines or 'Traditions' rather than being built out of rules or binding articles of association. The grassroots membership are involved in decision-making at all levels, and no clique can capture or subvert the operation to their ends or profit. Management is lean and low cost, and makes much use of voluntarism.

This chapter is centrally about therapeutic processes rather than management structures, but AA provides a case study in organisation that would repay the attention of any business school

AA and its relationship with the medical profession

Many AA members have achieved their recovery through the fellowship without any help from specialist treatment. To picture AA recovery as always an absolute and strict alternative to psychiatric involvement (or as antipathetic to medicine), would be false (Kurtz, 1985). Many drinkers will have found help both from AA and psychiatry, sequentially or at the same time. Medical practitioners have over many years shown an interest in AA (Williams, 1950, 1956) and provided facilities for AA meetings in hospital settings (Glatt, 1955), and AA has issued guidance on co-operation with the medical profession (Alcoholics Anonymous, 1955). Encouragement to attend AA given by a treatment agency can enhance attendance rates (Sisson and Mallams, 1991).

AA in support of natural processes of recovery

The preceding section has sought to describe the beliefs and operations of AA. Before trying to make any analysis of the inner therapeutic processes, one needs to try to understand what it will feel like to walk into the Thursday meeting at St Barnabas's Community Centre for the very first time, what it will mean to have a 'phone number in one's pocket and have that lifeline for use on a lonely weekend, what is implied in taking on the role of sponsor and testing oneself as someone who gives and knows what it means to be an AA member of 20 years' standing and yet be sober 'just for today', the excitement of a big event or a convention, AA as a transient and quickly rejected encounter or AA as a way of life. AA is a fellowship for the 'recovering alcoholic', for the drinker who is finding recovery hard going and who is drinking again next week, for the long-time sober member who has relapsed as well as being about 'contented sobriety'. There is no membership list and there is also no expulsion. Such is the mirror held up to nature.

Let's now turn to an examination of the varied, complex processes within the fellowship that may support recovery. The analysis should not be conducted in terms of a search for 'How uniquely does AA make people better?' Within the perspective of this chapter the question has rather to be 'How does AA assist different people in different ways, over time, toward a self-determined recovery?' In other words, what does AA offer toward support for natural processes of recovery?

Recovery may be aided by the unambiguous proximate, prioritised definition of goal

The person who arrives at his or her first AA meeting is likely, at the outset, to be muddled about the goal to aim for. Should the need to find a new job be put first, or should priority be given to dealing with debts, sorting out a fraught relationship or getting treatment for 'nerves', or should perhaps (only perhaps) priority attention be directed to stopping drinking and staying stopped?

In response to such confusion, AA offers a message on goal choice that is confident, unwavering, and hedged around with no provisos of any kind. AA will state that for the alcoholic, dealing with the drinking is the priority, and total abstinence (a day at a time), the only workable drinking goal.

In part speculatively but not without some support from research, one might infer that this unqualified insistence on abstinence is the crucial foundation for all else that AA offers toward enhancement of recovery. For the dependent drinker, return to controlled drinking is unlikely (Edwards *et al.*, 1983), and AA tends to attract dependent drinkers (Edwards *et al.*, 1987; Ogborne and Glaser, 1984). Without a personally defined and acceptable goal as alternative to temporising and makeshift stategies, the drinker is likely to go on moving in circles of relapse and reinstatement. The choice of an appropriate goal does not guarantee forward movement, but without acceptance of an abstinence goal, no constructive movement in most instances is likely to be achieved by the dependent drinker.

AA tends to present the 'one drink one drunk' postulate as proven and absolute truth rather than as statistically probable conjecture, and that declaration of certainty may alienate the research worker who knows that dependent drinkers often take an occasional drink without relapse, that partial relapse may be reversible before full relapse, and who will know that a percentage of heavy drinkers will in the long-term return to some kind of controlled drinking (Marlatt and Gordon, 1985). From the therapeutic perspective the question that has to be asked is whether AA's lack of equivocation or the research worker's honest airing of doubts is the more likely to assist the troubled dependent drinker. Many a liberal-minded therapist working in an alcoholism treatment centre would today talk about 'negotiation of goals' and would recoil from any proposal that they should impose the choice of goal. In reality the divide may not be absolute. AA well knows that it has no power to impose, but it does have the confidence (without negotiation) to propose.

If we take the task of this section as the attempt to discern what it is in AA that has made its message attractive to many people and which may speak to natural processes of recovery, consideration of the goal question and of the confidence with which that goal is stated must be the starting point. Perhaps the trouble drinker is often (but not always) best helped toward recovery by an acceptance of a goal that is an approximate truth and that is presented convincingly on a take it or leave it basis rather than by an honest prevarication. Perhaps at the start the conclusion to be drawn from the AA experience is that the professional therapist would do well to consider whether recovery from alcohol dependence is most often aided by entertaining complex alternatives, or by encouraging the personal admission of powerlessness over alcohol.

Recovery is made by motivation

If identification of a priority goal is the *sine qua non* for goal-directed change, there is then the question as to what factors are likely to support and sustain the individual's motivation in striving toward the chosen goal. Motivation is a complex psychological concept that has been discussed within a number of psychological models (see Chapters 11 and 12).

Motivation can, for instance, be seen as determined by the individual's integration of the field of negative and positive consequences that will attach to a certain course of action (or to not taking that action). The individual is situated in a pay-off matrix that has as its framework the consequences of actions and inactions, coloured and interpreted by a subjective appraisal of the likelihood of any eventuality, and the personal value to be placed on any consequence (Orford, 1977). Another approach to the psychology of motivation emphasises the importance of personal belief in the capacity to change, or self-efficacy (Bandura 1982; Sutton, 1987). Within that view, drinkers must believe that they are potential winners and have it within them to achieve the abstinence goal, otherwise there is no motivation to try for that goal.

How may AA be able to bolster motivation? Let's examine that question within a combined model that puts the individual's belief in ability to effect change within the pay-off matrix that calculates the profit and loss of change. As regards enhancement of belief in self-efficacy, the person who comes to an AA meeting will hear and see people who manifestly speak to the fact that sobriety is achievable. Some may be talking about success in the first weeks of struggle and thus offer immediate, empathetic possibilities of identification, and their statements may be more pertinent to the newcomer than the Olympian achievements of the evening's chairman who is talking about his or her 10 years without a drink. Furthermore, and with what might be seen as brilliant sleight of hand, AA bolsters self-efficacy by insisting that the goal for everyone (even the ten-year sober chairman), is the simple, proximal and not too daunting task of staying sober 'just for today'. The tactics are to make goal-directed achievement seem disarmingly possible by minimalising the size of the task.

As regards AA's influence on the individual's appraisal of the personal pay-offs, the AA meeting, the sponsor, the AA culture, will all repeatedly and insistently carry the message that sobriety will bring personal benefit, and drinking disbenefit. Again through role-modelling, these messages are carried not only in words but more tangibly. The speaker who been sober for a few months says that it is good to wake up looking forward to the day rather than retching and sweating and searching for the bottle, and beyond the words he or she seems to have the appearance of someone who is enjoying each day as it comes. Material goods as well as psychological health can carry conviction and feed into the pay-off calculus, and someone whose drinking had a few months ago brought them to sleeping on the street is tonight wearing a rather good suit. There is the likelihood that within the roomful of people something will be said that causes the person who is taking the first steps toward sobriety to say 'That might be me', and in consequence shift his or her estimate of the pay-offs toward a positive balance. AA thus offers strong reinforcement for a positive view of the benefits that will accrue from sobriety. But with the background message also that 'alcoholism is a progressive disease' (Durand, 1994) and that with continued drinking life will only get worse still, there is at the same time the consistent invitation to weight drinking negatively.

Something else to do

For the dependent drinker, drinking will often have become a dominant time commitment. There is always somewhere to go (the pub or the bar) and something to do (drink). The friendship circle is likely to be progressively narrowed to a circle of drinking companions, and they will provide a ready source of human contact, however superficial. And life has purpose, which is to obtain the price of the next drink. There is no sense of time hanging heavily.

With drink surrendered, the question of what can substitute for the time-filling, companion-providing, purpose-defining aspects of alcohol becomes pressingly apparent. What can take its place? Research both from the USA (Vaillant, 1983) and the UK (Edwards *et al.*, 1992) shows that recovery from alcohol dependence is often related to the individual's discovery of rewardingness. AA puts on offer much that is potentially responsive to this kind of need. One meeting will fill only a few hours of a single evening, but the person who is coming new to AA will be encouraged to attend '90 meetings in 90 days', and there are daytime as well as evening meetings. In addition to meetings there are all those types of activities that can go on outside the meetings (p. 228). Furthermore, AA does not offer just a passive time-filler, but the possibility of an active engagement in new and rewarding patterns of life.

The skills to work recovery

Supposing that the individual has defined abstinence as the goal and is motivated to pursue that goal, there is still then the question of how they are going to equip themselves effectively and practically to take on the tasks inherent to achieving the goal. Many aspects of AA activity seem designed to teach the necessary cognitive and coping skills for achievement and maintenance of the drink-free life. Indeed, an AA meeting can sometimes seem almost to take on the guise of a cognitive-behavioural workshop. Don't get tired, don't get angry, learn to laugh at yourself, see the other person's point of view. Look out for the tricks your thinking can play on you, the planned relapse, the planned excuses, the self-justifying resentments. Have something else to do, don't get bored. Carry some chocolate. Count your blessings. Don't go to that party if you are going to find the temptation to drink too great.

Thus a great deal of what psychologists have written from the theoretical and research point of view regarding the cognitions and coping skills that support the recovery process, are the everyday stuff of AA wisdom (DiClemente, 1993; Morgenstern and McCrady, 1993). Recovery, AA appears to tell us, is partly about learning some simple ways of seeing oneself and others and situations differently, and is also about having the skills to react differently to situations that would in the past have cued drinking. Solid recovery is about incremental practice of these skills.

Questions about the spiritual dimension

Spirituality has been described by Miller (1990) as 'the silent dimension in addiction research'. AA challenges the academic community to think more openly about the significance of spirituality in recovery from alcohol dependence (Garsuch, 1993). There are likely to be problems for the scientist in agreeing an operational definition of what is to be meant by the spiritual dimension, and some fear that the attempt to define may all too easily be tainted by reductionism, and pass by the essence (Spilka *et al.*, 1985). A scale is available for the measurement of spirituality (Garsuch., 1988), and it has been employed in alcohol research. AA, it has been suggested, is not a self-help programme, but a God-help programme (Kurtz, 1993).

The emphasis on God to be found in the Twelve Steps has been discussed earlier (p. 224), and the suggestion was made that the interpretation given to the concept of 'higher power' can be very personal, even atheistical. Nonetheless, several authorities have recently given support to Miller's contention that spirituality is something with which research workers should now reckon. The suggestion has been made that AA may operate through a spiritual force, and that spirituality is the unique ingredient of the fellowship's success (Garsuch, 1993).

As ever, it is likely that different people will gain different things from AA. Some will find it a non-denominational religion with which they are more at ease than they were with the religion of their upbringing. Others will return through AA to reconciliation with religion. Research does, however, suggest that at least in the UK, the religious element in AA is not rated as the dominantly helpful factor in what AA gives to its members. An 'Attributions Inventory' was completed by 62 male alcoholics at the ten-year point in a follow-up study (Edwards *et al.*, 1987). Not all these subjects had ever attempted AA or affiliated to it with any intensity. Overall results showed that 32% of the sample rated positively 'Hearing other people's stories at AA', 25% 'Friendship through AA', 24% 'Going to AA a lot', 18% 'Telling own story at AA'. The lowest scoring item in this set, at 7%, was 'The religious element in AA'.

One study based on limited sampling should not be over-interpreted, and different results might have been obtained with other samples or in another country. Perhaps in this instance what we should most learn from AA is that the natural path to recovery for one person may not be so natural to another. AA offers access to spiritual experience for those who want, when they want it.

Learning from AA

AA is not a repository to be picked through clumsily by this or that therapist or theoretician keen to bolster the credibility of their special practice approach or view of the world. It is a phenomenon that should be approached respectfully (Kurtz, 1993). Respect does not, however, require adulation. It should be admitted that we still know little or nothing about whether AA is effective within the terms that would be expected of a controlled trial (Bebbington, 1976; Glaser and Ogborne, 1982; Ogborne, 1989, 1993). To pin that model of evaluation on AA may, though, to an extent be inappropriate and randomisation may not be a feasible research design, although it has been attempted (Ditman *et al.*, 1967; Brandsma *et al.*, 1980; Walsh *et al.*, 1991). But whatever our admiration for AA as naturalistic phenomenon, we should not lose sight of the fact that, to date, the evidence for efficacy is very incomplete. Many people who go to AA will drop out after one or two meetings (Miller and McCrady, 1993). The message of total abstinence will not be helpful to the majority of excessive drinkers who are encountered in the primary care setting. Put simply, the evidence that AA 'works' is suggestive and rests on the evidence for its popularity and seeming ability to meet need, rather than being a matter of proven fact. AA does not help everyone, and refusal to attend is not tantamount to 'denial'.

If we concede that adulation is likely to be unhelpful, there is then the still respectful question as to what may reasonably be learnt by the professional from the complex totality of the AA experience (Edwards, 1964). What happens when people with drinking problems come together and design their own recovery programme, building on experience, felt need, trial and error, what goes on in the church hall, rather than being governed by the professional world?

That question is, of course, central to the purpose of this chapter. If AA holds up a mirror to the natural process of recovery, what do we now see in that mirror? What that mirror seems most clearly to show is that recovery is an active, doing, process, rather than a conversation in a room. It is a process rather than an event. Recovery is about what people do for themselves rather than what is done for them or to them. It is about finding an acceptable personal goal, enhancing motivation, learning recovery skills, and finding positive substitutes for drinking. It is about stopping drinking, but it is also about more than that. For some people recovery is about finding a way to God, while probably for others it may be important to make the discovery that it is possible to be sober and happy with doubt, or atheism.

None of this is to suggest surrender to nature worship, an anti-intellectual view, or the pretence that AA has everything to teach us with the hard-won scientific base discarded. But it is to argue that in designing treatment programmes, practising treatment, and researching treatment efficacy, the professional may do well to heed nature, with AA a reflecting mirror.

References

Alcoholics Anonymous (1952) *Twelve Steps and Twelve Traditions*: New York: Alcoholics Anonymous World Service.

Alcoholics Anonymous (1955) *Alcoholics Anonymous and the Medical Profession*. New York: AA World Service Inc.

Alcoholics Anonymous (1976) *Alcoholics Anonymous: The Story of How Many Thousands of Men and Women Have Recovered From Alcoholism*. York, NJ: AA General Services Office.

Alcoholics Anonymous (1990) *World Headquarters 1989 Membership Survey*. New York: AA World Service.

Bacon, S. D. (1957) A sociological look at AA. *Minnesota Welfare*, **10**, 35–44.

Bales, R. F. (1944) The therapeutic role of 'Alcoholics Anonymous' as seen by a sociologist. *Quarterly Journal of Studies on Alcohol*, **5**, 267–78.

Bandura, A. (1982) Self efficacy mechanisms in human agency. *American Psychologist*, **37**, 122–47.

Bebbington, P. E. (1976) The efficacy of Alcoholics Anonymous: the elusiveness of hard data. *British Journal of Psychiatry*, **128**, 572–80.

Brandsma, J. M., Maultsby, M. C. and Walsh, R. J. (1980) *Outpatient Treatment of Alcoholism: A Review and Comparative Study*. Baltimore, Md. University Park Press.

Cook, C. H. (1988a) The Minnesota model in the management of drug and alcohol dependency. Part I. *British Journal of Addiction*, **83**, 625–34.

Cook, C. H. (1988b) The Minnesota model in the management of drug and alcohol dependency. Part II. *British Journal of Addiction*, **83**, 735–48.

Cooper, J. and Maule, H. G. (1962) Problems of drinking: an enquiry among members of 'Alcoholics Anonymous'. *British Journal of Addiction*, **58**, 45–53.

DiClemente, C. (1993) Alcoholics Anonymous and the structure of change. In: McCrady, B. S. and Miller, W. R. (eds.) *Research on Alcoholics Anonymous, Opportunities and Alternatives*, pp. 79–97. New Brunswick NJ: Rutgers Center of Alcohol Studies.

Ditman, K. S., Crawford, G. G., Forgy, E. W. and Moskowitz, H. (1967) A controlled experiment on the use of court probation for drunk arrests. *American Journal of Psychiatry*, **124**, 160–3.

Durand, M. A. (1994) The image of 'progressive disease'. In: Edwards, G. and Lader, M. (eds.) *Addiction: Processes of Change*, pp. 95–110. Oxford: Oxford University Press.

Edwards, G. (1964) The puzzle of AA. *New Society*, 28th May.

Edwards, G. (1987) Alcoholics Anonymous. In: Edwards, G. (ed.) *The Treatment of Drinking Problems*, 2nd edn, pp. 257–65. Oxford: Blackwell Scientific.

Edwards, G., Brown, D., Duckitt, A., Oppenheimer, E., Sheehan, M. and Taylor, C. (1987) Outcome of alcoholism: the structure of patient attribution as to what causes change. *British Journal of Addiction*, **82**, 533–45.

Edwards, G., Duckitt, A., Oppenheimer, E., Sheehan, M. and Taylor, C. (1983) What happens to alcoholics? *Lancet* **ii**, 269–71.

Edwards, G., Hensman, C., Hawker, A. and Williamson, V. (1967) Alcoholics Anonymous: the anatomy of a self-help group. *Social Psychiatry*, **1**, 195–204.

Edwards, G., Oppenheimer, E. and Taylor, C. (1992) Hearing the noise in the system. Exploration of textual analysis as a method for studying change in drinking behaviour. *British Journal of Addiction*, **87**, 73–81.

Fowler, W. J. (1993) Alcoholics Anonymous and faith development. In: McCrady, B. S. and Miller, W. R. (eds.) *Research on Alcoholics Anonymous, Opportunities and Alternatives*, pp. 113–35. New Brunswick, NJ: Rutgers Center of Alcohol Studies.

Garsuch, R. L. (1988) The psychology of religion. *Annual Review of Psychology*, **39**, 201–11.

Garsuch, R. L. (1993) Assessing spiritual variables in Alcoholics Anonymous research. In: McCrady, B. S. and Miller,W. R. (eds.) *Research on Alcoholics Anonymous, Opportunities and Alternatives*, pp. 301–18. Brunswick NJ, Rutgers Center of Alcohol Studies.

Glaser, F. B. and Ogborne, A. C. (1982) Does AA really work? *British Journal of Addiction*, **77**, 123–9.

Glatt, M. M. (1955) A treatment centre for alcoholics. *British Journal of Addiction*, **52**, 55–89.

Kurtz, L. F. (1985) Co-operation and rivalry between helping professionals and members of AA. *Health and Social Work*, **10**, 104–12.

Kurtz, E. (1993) Research on Alcoholics Anonymous: the historical context. In: McCrady, B. S. and Miller, W. R. (eds.) *Research on Alcoholics Anonymous, Opportunities and Alternatives*, pp. 13–26. New Brunswick, NJ: Rutgers Center of Alcohol Studies.

Mäkelä, K. (1991) Social and cultural preconditions of Alcoholics Anonymous (AA) and factors associated with the strength of AA. *British Journal of Addiction*, **86**, 1405–13.

Marlatt, G. A. and Gordon, J. R. (1985) *Relapse Prevention: Maintenance Strategies in the Treatment of Addictive Behaviours*. New York: Guilford Press.

McCrady, B. S. and Miller, W. R. (eds.) (1993) *Research on Alcoholics Anonymous, Opportunities and Alternatives*. New Brunswick, NJ: Rutgers Center of Alcohol Studies.

Miller, W. R. (1990) Spirituality: The silent dimension in addiction research. *Drug and Alcohol Review*, **9**, 259–66.

Miller, W. R. and McCrady, B. S. (1993) The importance of research in
    Alcoholics Anonymous. In: McCrady, B. S. and Miller, W. R. (eds.)
    Research on Alcoholics Anonymous, Opportunities and Alternatives, pp. 3–
    11. New Brunswick, NJ: Rutgers Center of Alcohol Studies.
Morgenstern, J. and McCrady B. S. (1993) Cognitive processes and change in
    disease model treatment. In: McCrady, B. S. and Miller, W. R. (eds.)
    Research on Alcoholics Anonymous, Opportunities and Alternatives, pp.
    153–64. New Brunswick, NJ: Rutgers Center of Alcohol Studies.
Ogborne, A. C. (1989) Some limitations of Alcoholics Anonymous. In:
    Galanter, M. (ed.) *Recent Development in Alcoholism Vol. 7, Treatment
    Research*. New York: Plenum.
Ogborne, A. C. (1993) Assessing the effectiveness of Alcoholics Anonymous:
    meeting the challenges. In: McCrady, B. S. and Miller, W. R. (eds.)
    Research on Alcoholics Anonymous, Opportunities and Alternatives, pp.
    339–55. New Brunswick NJ: Rutgers Center of Alcohol Studies.
Ogborne, A. C. and Glaser, F. B. (1984) Characteristics of affiliates of
    Alcoholics Anonymous. *Journal of Studies on Alcohol*, **42**, 661–75.
Orford, J. (1977) What psychology offers. In: Edwards, G. and Grant, M.
    (eds.) *Alcoholism: New Knowledge and New Responses*, pp. 88–89. London:
    Croon Helm.
Orford, J. and Edwards, G. (1977) *Alcoholism. A Comparison of Treatment and
    Advice, with a Study of the Influence of Marriage*. Maudsley Monograph
    26. Oxford: Oxford University Press.
Robinson, D. (1979) *Talking Out of Alcoholism. The Self-help process of
    Alcoholics Anonymous*. London: Croon Helm.
Robinson, D. and Henry, S. (1977) *Self-Help and Health: Mutual Aid for
    Modern Problems*. London: Martin Robertson.
Room, R. (1993) Alcoholics Anonymous as a social movement. In: McCrady,
    B. S. and Miller, W. R. (eds.) *Research on Alcoholics Anonymous,
    Opportunities and Alternatives*, pp. 167–87. New Brunswick NJ: Rutgers
    Center of Alcohol Studies.
Sisson, R. and Mallams, T. H. (1991) The use of systematic encouragement
    and community access procedures to increase attendance at Alcoholics
    Anonymous and Al-Anon meetings. *American Journal of Drug and Alcohol
    Abuse*, **8**, 371–6.
Spilka, B., Hood, R. W. and Gorsuch, R. L. (1985) *The Psychology of
    Religion: An Empirical Approach*. Englewood Cliffs, NJ: Prentice-Hall.
Sutton, S. R. (1987) Social psychological approaches to understanding
    addiction behaviour. *British Journal of Addiction*, **82**, 355–70.
Tiebout, H. M. (1944) Therapeutic mechanisms of Alcoholics Anonymous.
    American Journal of Psychiatry, **100**, 468–73.
Tiebout, H. M. (1953) Surrender vs. compliance in therapy with special
    reference to alcoholism. *Quarterly Journal of Studies on Alcohol*, **110**,
    48–58.
Vaillant, G. E. (1980) The Doctor's Dilemma. In: Edwards, G. and Grant, M.
    (eds.) *Alcoholism Treatment in Transition*, pp. 13–31. London: Croon
    Helm.
Vaillant, G. E. (1983) *The Natural History of Alcoholism*. Cambridge: Harvard
    University Press.

Walsh, D. C., Hingson, R. W., Merrigan, D. M. and Levenson, S. M. (1991) A randomized trial of treatment options for alcohol abusing workers. *New England Journal of Medicine*, **325**, 775–8.

Williams, L. (1950) Some observations on the recent advances in the treatment of alcoholism. *British Journal of Addiction*, **47**, 62–7.

Williams, L. (1956) *Alcoholism: A Manual for Students and Practitioners.* Edinburgh: E. and S. Livingstone.

15

How therapeutic communities work

KINGSLEY NORTON

The concept and its definition

The term therapeutic community was coined by Lt Colonel Tom Main, RAMC in 'The hospital as a therapeutic instition' (Main, 1946). Later he referred to the therapeutic community as a 'culture of enquiry . . . into personal and interpersonal and intersystem problems and a study of impulses, defences, and relations as these are expressed and arranged socially' (Main, 1983). In the same paper he acknowledged that the term therapeutic community owed most of its meaning to Maxwell Jones whose 'innovative work, especially wth psychopaths at the Social Rehabilitation Unit of Belmont Hospital (now called Henderson Hospital) and voluminous writings about his own percepts and practices have much influenced others'. The following extracts from the work of Tom Main (Main, 1946) and Maxwell Jones (Jones, 1952, 1956, 1968), illustrate some of their respective pioneering contributions to the concept of therapeutic community, which are still pertinent to current clinical practice.

Main referred to the therapeutic community as 'an attempt to use a hospital not as an organisation run by doctors in the interests of their own greater technical efficiency, but as a community with the immediate aim of full participation of all its members in its daily life with the eventual aim of re-socialisation of the neurotic individual for life in ordinary society'. He continued that it should be, ideally, 'a spontaneous and emotionally structured organisation rather than one which is medically dictated'. He stressed 'the importance of the daily life of the therapeutic community being related to real tasks, i.e. those which are truly relevant to the needs and aspirations of the small society of the hospital, together with the larger society in which it is set'. He acknowledged that these were 'not small requirements . . . [and that they] demanded a

240

review of our own attitudes as psychiatrists towards our own status and responsibilities'. One result was that the doctor would no longer be seen, and would not see himself or herself, as owning patients. Rather, the patients would be 'given up to the community which is to treat them and [which] owns him and them'. Thus, 'patients are no longer captive children, obedient in nursery-like activities, but have sincere adult roles to play and are free to reach for responsibilities and opinions concerning the community of which they are a part . . . Failures of organisation, internal problems of apathy, insecurity and hostility, as well as ordinary practical difficulties are matters for solution by the patients who own the community and create the problems'.

Jones wrote along very similar lines, hence 'Therapeutic community implies that the responsibility for treatment is not confined to the trained medical staff but is also the concern of other community members, i.e. the patients'. He recognised the importance of staff tensions as they affect the treatment of patients in their charge, and discussed the limitations of construing patients in hospital solely in 'individual dynamic-historical terms'. He argued that patient groups, lacking an adequate channel of communication to the staff, protected themselves by turning inwards and developing a social structure that was insulated as much as possible from the friction of the hospital routine. Such friction, he believed, led to behaviour on the part of the patients that, although resembling neurotic behaviour arising from personal emotional conflicts, was in fact to a considerable extent due to factors in the immediate situation, that is, those to which staff also contributed.

Jones emphasised how far traditional staff and patient roles needed revision in order to facilitate the active participation of patients and the development of a truly therapeutic community and summarised the situation thus:

1. Treatment is a continuous process throughout the working life of the patient and reactions to hospital are similar to those which obtain outside of it, therefore their study provides useful information regarding patients' existential problems.
2. The above requires reorganisation of the hospital structure, including more open communication, less rigid hierarchy between doctor/nurse/patients, and daily discussions of the whole unit and its sub-groups.
3. The above necessarily leads to a reappraisal of the place of the patient in the social structure of the hospital.

Therapeutic community 'approach' versus therapeutic community 'proper'

Some writers have distinguished between what is referred to as a therapeutic community approach and therapeutic community proper (for example, Clarke, 1965). The main differences are summarised in Table 15.1 (after Manning, 1989).

Therapeutic community proper – democratic style

The therapeutic community proper, otherwise referred to as a democratic style therapeutic community, is based on the model developed by Maxwell Jones. At Henderson Hospital, one example of a democratic style therapeutic community, all treatments are in a group setting (with

Table 15.1 *Types of therapeutic community*

Therapeutic community approach	Therapeutic community proper
Acute admissions service	No acute admission service
Catchment area from which most patients are drawn	No catchment area
Does not specialise in certain disorders/problems	Does specialise – favours neurotic/personality disorders over psychotics
Majority of patients are non-residential	Majority of patients are residential
Patients generally older (40 years)	Patients generally young (most in their 20s)
Most referrals from GPs	Most referrals from psychiatrists, special units, social services, etc.
Most referrers have no alternative place to refer	Most referrers could have referred elsewhere
Higher number of referrals (400 – 600 + p.a.)	Lower number of referrals (200 – 300 p.a.)
Does not encourage or discourage referrals	Does tend to encourage and discourage referrals

the exception of a GP surgery function, which is carried out by medical and nursing staff from within the hospital). The emphasis is on socio-dynamic exploration of patients' social actions through confrontation by fellow patients and staff, and by psychodynamic exploration of patients' feelings through interpretation by the psychotherapist (Whiteley, 1986). Sociotherapy and psychotherapy are not viewed as competing treatment ingredients but as having a summative effect, particularly when used 'in phase' (Edelson, 1970).

Clientele

The main application of the hospital-based democratic therapeutic community approach has been to seriously neurotic or personality-disordered individuals. Henderson Hospital has a population of moderately to severely personality-disordered adult patients (known as residents), in the age range 17 to 45. In DSM-III-R Axis 2 diagnostic terms (APA, 1987) they come from all three clusters of personality disorder sub-type but especially from cluster B, i.e. histrionic, narcissistic, antisocial and borderline personality disorder. Considered in terms of presenting symptoms and behaviours, they provide a wide range (see Figures 15.1 and 15.2). Many have been treated with psychotropic medication and ECT in the past, but at Henderson Hospital no psychotropic medication is prescribed and the task confronting the residents is to acquire and maintain human, rather than chemical, support.

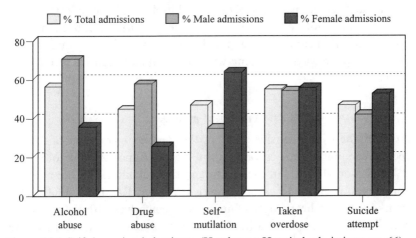

Figure 15.1 Self-damaging behaviours (Henderson Hospital admissions, $n = 66$).

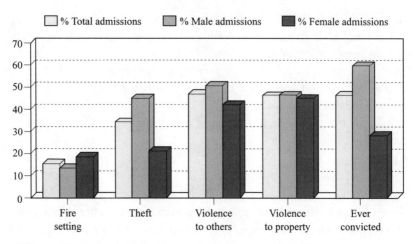

Figure 15.2 Antisocial behaviours (Henderson Hospital admissions, $n = 66$).

Usually the community comprises roughly equal numbers of men and women, up to a total of 29. The vast majority are single and the average age is approximately 25. The average length of stay is seven months with a maximum of one year. Many residents (approximately 25%) are unable to make the difficult adjustment to living in the therapeutic community; they leave prematurely because yielding up their habitual means of reducing anxiety and psychic pain, especially those involving acting out behaviours (including violence to self, others or property or the misuse of drugs and alcohol), is hard to do. Acceptance for admission by the community, and the admission to the hospital itself, imply accepting a treatment contract not to indulge in such behaviours, and beginning to depend on verbal communication and exploration to identify and change the maladaptive ways of dealing with powerful and negative feelings.

Treatment process

Probably the most intensive study of the treatment processes of a therapeutic community was carried out by Robert Rapoport and colleagues at Henderson Hospital in the 1950s, and this culminated in the publication of a book entitled *The Community as Doctor* (Rapoport, 1960). This team of social anthropologists familiarised themselves with the unit for a year before studying, over a further number of years, the ideology of the unit, in terms of the belief systems held by staff and the social structure and processes operative within the unit. Perhaps reflecting their anthropological background, the team saw ideas and cultural themes as being central to understanding the cohesion of the unit, and they identified three propositions held by staff, which they felt were fundamental: 'Everything is treatment'; 'All treatment is rehabilitation'; and 'All patients (once admitted) should get the same treatment'.

The team also identified four cultural themes that were thought to underlay the above propositions:

1. 'Democratisation': referring to the unit's view that each member of the community should share equally in the exercise of power in decision-making about community affairs, both therapeutic and administrative, and the belief that the conventional hospital hierarchies should be 'flattened' to produce a more egalitarian form of participation.
2. 'Permissiveness': referring to the unit's belief that it should function with all its members tolerating from one another a wide degree of behaviour that might be distressing or seem deviant according to 'ordinary' norms. Ideally, this should allow both for individuals freely to expose their behavioural dificulties, and for others to react freely to this so that the bases for both sides of social relationship patterns can be examined.
3. 'Communalism': referring to the unit's belief that its functioning should be characterised by inter-communicative and intimate sets of relationships. Sharing of amenities, informality (for instance, use of first names), and 'freeing' communication are prescribed. (NB 'Freeing' refers to the open and direct, hence free, expression of feelings by all members of the community – residents and staff. This is held to foster beneficial improvement, over the practices of more conventional hospitals, to the administrative aspects of the life of the therapeutic community as well as providing a cathartic function for the individuals concerned).
4. 'Reality confrontation': referring to the unit's belief that patients should be continuously presented with interpretations of their behaviour as it is seen by most others. This is meant to counteract patients' tendencies to use massive denial, distortion, withdrawal, or other mechanisms that interfere with their capacity to relate to others in the normal world.

Whiteley (Medical Director of Henderson Hospital for 22 years, until 1989) characterised the treatment process by three modes, which to some extent also represent three sequential stages, within treatment – interaction, exploration and experimentation (Whiteley, 1986). Interaction and exploration are facilitated by the large number of rules in the community that serve to maximise attendance at group meetings (thereby ensuring interaction in those residents who would otherwise seek to avoid social contact). These rules also minimise acting out by setting up emergency meetings to examine attitudes and feelings, ideally before these have spilled over into action (see below). Through experimentation the individual resident tries out other modes of coping.

Engagement in therapy

Regardless of the treatment method or setting, regular difficulties are encountered in treating personality-disordered patients. Problems centre on their meaningful engagement and continuing in therapy. A feature of the Henderson Hospital model is that treatment is voluntary, and never a direct condition of a criminal court disposal. Residents are not admitted under Sections of the Mental Health Act (1983).

Facilitating engagement is a paramount concern and the process of engagement begins at the patient's selection interview. As with all Henderson activities, selection is made in a group setting by residents and staff together (an example of 'communalism'). Residents outnumber staff by between two and three to one. Three candidates for admission are invited to each selection group interview and are interviewed, sequentially, by the group. Candidates are invited to talk about: themselves as people; their current and past difficulties; previous treatment received; aspects of their childhood and adolescence; and they are asked what problems they would wish to address if admitted to Henderson. Notes relating to the interviews are taken by one staff and one resident member, and the latter's record of the interview is presented to the whole community prior to a successful candidate's admission.

After the formal group interview, there is a closed discussion of the candidates, by staff and residents. This culminates in a democratic vote, for or against the admission of each candidate. Residents can readily out-vote staff and thus they have the major say in who is admitted (an example of 'democratisation').

Of the residents, only the more senior (longer than three months' experience of Henderson's treatment) are involved in the selection process, which itself is an important ingredient of their own treatment. During the selection group, these residents experience the weight of decision-making, being on the 'authority' end of the transaction, for a change, and potentially saying 'no' as well as 'yes' to a candidate's request for admission. Residents see themselves and their difficulties reflected in the candidates who come for admission, and they begin to realise how they appear to others or how they used to appear. Heated discussion often results over whether or not to admit, particularly when there are issues of sexual victimisation, physical violence, arson, homosexuality, or racial prejudice. All of this is grist to the therapeutic mill of the community.

Research into the selection process, using SCL-90R (Derogatis *et al.*, 1973) has shown that those not selected (approximately one-third of candidates interviewed) tend to be more somatising, obsessive-compulsive and phobic in their symptomatology (Dolan *et al.*, 1990). It appears, therefore, that the selection group is choosing those who have a capacity to verbalise feelings and psychosocial difficulties, and to function in a group setting. The latter is important since all therapy is group-based, from the daily community meeting (involving all residents and staff), through to the small group psychotherapy (thrice weekly), to art therapy, psychodrama (both weekly events), and the task-centred work groups (cookery, gardening and maintenance, and artwork, each twice weekly).

Even when meaningful engagement has been established, remaining in treatment long enough to make lasting personality change is problematic. At Henderson, keeping engaged in therapy is facilitated via a variety of features in the hospital's internal organisation and operation, resulting in a therapeutic blend of supportive containment and confrontation.

Formal patient hierarchy

The resident group, as a whole, is deliberately hierarchically structured, with respect to elected positions or jobs within the community that residents hold for a month at a time. Changing post-holders means that residents gain experience of being on both ends of a responsibility and authority spectrum. The posts relate to actual tasks that need to be carried out for the internal running of the unit, both within unstructured time and the formal treatment programme. The accent, however, is on how the task is undertaken, and on 'means' rather then 'ends' (Norton, 1990).

The community is headed by the 'Top Three' residents who are supported by a fourth, the 'General Secretary'. These four residents, who have to have been resident for at least three months in order to be nominated for election to their positions, co-ordinate the main day-to-day community activities during the one month's tenure of their posts. This includes the important roles of: (1) setting the agenda for the day's community meeting at a 10 p.m. meeting, called the 'Summit', the previous evening; (2) chairing the daily community meeting (9.15–10.30 a.m.); (3) leading the weekly selection group; and (4) deciding on the need to call emergency meetings of the community, in the face of a major incident or problem within the community.

Other elected posts are open to residents, again on the basis of seniority (length of stay within Henderson) and include among others: keeping of a daily register of residents' attendance at therapy groups, cooking and storage of food, and devising cleaning rotas. There are sufficient jobs for all residents. In the monthly elections to these posts only residents are able to vote on the nominations, although staff participate in the discussions prior to the voting.

One of the larger gaps between the levels in the resident's hierarchical organisation is that between 'new' residents and the remainder. 'New' residents have a three-week induction period, including their own small group, and enjoy a privileged position by virtue of being excused cleaning duties during their first week. However, 'new' residents are not allowed to vote in the first week and are therefore more to be seen than heard in the community. The 'new' resident may test his or her position in the pecking order, often via rule-breaking, for example bringing alcohol or illicit drugs into the hospital. This will provide an insight into how the rules of the community are implemented (see below). One effect of the hierarchical organisation is that residents know where they stand in the formal hierarchy and, overall, this can facilitate a feeling of security or containment. For many residents this forms a marked contrast to their family of origin, wherein parent–child boundaries and responsibilities were blurred or otherwise eroded or breached.

Rigid timetable

Containment is also effected via the community's rigidly organised programme of therapy with fixed time boundaries, strictly adhered to, albeit with fixed periods of leeway. Thus ten minutes' absence from a therapy group is the maximum amount that is tolerated by the community. If more than that is missed, the group is officially missed and recorded as such. The fact of this is then routinely announced at the next day's community meeting, under one of the standing items of the agenda, and the resident in question has to account for the absence. Missing more than two therapy groups in one week means that all groups the next day must be attended in full and, at the end of this, a treatability vote is taken by the whole community to decide whether the resident in question should be discharged or remain in treatment. Again, residents' greater numbers mean that they have the greater power to decide on who leaves and when. The resident in question will be discharged from the community unless an adequate reason, show of remorse, or good intentions for the future, results and is accepted. Given that a second admission to Henderson is unlikely, discharge is the ultimate censure whose power, of course, depends on the resident being sufficiently engaged with the community.

Those who are not prematurely discharged become increasingly attached to the community and its members. Because of the variety in the structured programme, and the large amount of social contact that takes place in the unstructured time (including during the undertaking of domestic duties), there are many niches into which individual residents may fit with a beneficial impact on self-esteem (Norris, 1983). Some tasks demand more verbal skills and others more practical or manual ones.

Rules: breaking and enforcing

The more serious rules, to do with proscribing violence (to self, others and property), and drug and alcohol misuse, occasion automatic discharge when broken. The rule-breaker is considered by the community to have self-discharged, but he or she may ask for permission to stay on the unit until the community meets in full the following morning (an example of 'permissiveness' and of tolerance of greater deviance than is normal in society at large). Assuming permission is granted (via a decision of all members of the community, following discussion at an emergency meeting), that person has to attend all therapy groups the following day and then undergo a 'readmission' vote.

Perhaps it is surprising that enforcing the community's rules at Henderson is relatively easy. The major reason is that it is primarily the residents themselves who enforce the rules. Rule enforcement by residents who have been on the receiving end of intoxicated, disordered, violent, neglectful or abusing authority figures previously in their lives, provides important empowerment to people who more often have been disempowered victims. However, the tendency is towards a harsh, unempathic and unthinking rule enforcement, and staff need to act to mitigate this effect (Norton, 1992).

Community meeting

The morning (Monday to Saturday) community meeting is crucial. It is a forum for all residents and all staff on duty to meet and to discuss matters of relevance to the community as a whole. The meeting has a number of standing items as well as a more open part of the agenda. It is chaired, in rotation, by the 'Top Three' residents. Missing the community meeting, or more than ten minutes of it, results in automatic 'assessment' – having to attend all therapy groups the following day and then to face a treatability vote as described above.

The meeting deals with most of the day-to-day administrative activity associated with running the community, for example, co-ordinating cooking, washing up, and handover meetings. At a given item on the agenda, staff are invited to feedback matters concerning, for example, annual leave, writing of reports, and any nursing or medical matters. Residents' minutes are presented from a 'wind-down' meeting, which is held each evening at 9.15 p.m., for those who for one reason or another are finding it difficult to settle for the night. Matters arising, together with any other topics identified by the 'Top Three' as being of importance to the community at the time, appear as standing items on the next morning's agenda. In this way topical issues, for example the community's upset after a resident has been discharged (which otherwise might be ignored or denied), are brought to the attention of the community as a whole. Personality clashes or other problems between residents, or between residents and staff, are discussed and potentially resolved in this setting. The meeting serves directly or indirectly many important functions, including enhancing the cohesion and a feeling of belonging to the community, alerting the community's attention to its distressed members, and executing an examination of rule-breaking behaviour. Most of the 'votes' are carried out in this setting (see above).

Response to serious incidents or distress

Having become engaged in treatment, residents struggle to keep to the rules of the community but inevitably these get broken. If an important rule (one occasioning automatic discharge) has been broken, or a resident is particularly distressed, and a discussion of this cannot wait until the next day's community meeting, the 'Top Three' residents will call an emergency meeting at any time of day or night. All community members must attend or else face a discharge vote themselves. The various human resources of the community may be mobilised in order to support the resident in question. At night, this may entail others sleeping in or outside the individual's bedroom, or a number of residents, together with the distressed person, occupying a large room with their mattresses. No psychotropic medication is prescribed.

There is much emotional and practical support in the community for those residents viewed by their peers as being deserving, and especially for those who have previously provided such support for others or who are viewed as 'really working' on their problems. Tolerance, however, is limited and this fact can be beneficial, often resulting in confrontation over the distressed role having been overplayed and having turned into an act of manipulation – if your fellow residents have repeatedly sat up with you through the night, they will not be pleased if you fail to mend your deviant ways of expressing distress and will recommend that you start to use the therapy groups during daylight hours. Thus, compared to many other settings, deviant behaviour as a way of expressing otherwise unbearable psychic pain is not reinforced, whereas genuine struggling with emotion is. There is no 'specialling' by staff and therefore no seemingly endless supply of one-to-one professional relationships, which can tend to reinforce sick, or manipulative, behaviour.

Disengaging

For those who stay, Henderson has often become a place of special attachment and security, and leaving it is difficult. For some residents their experience of leaving has been synonymous with that of expulsion or other traumatic separation and often the community will be set up by such a resident in order for this pattern to be repeated. Regressed rule-breaking, reminiscent of the resident's earlier stages of treatment, is frequently the form in which testing out takes place, and there is no shortage of rules to break. Once this strategy is seen through, however, the resident is supported, encouraged, cajoled or shamed by the community into owning his or her feelings in the face of leaving, which then becomes an important part of working through leaving. Anger is often an easier emotion to tolerate than sadness and also a camouflage for sadness and the pain of leaving. Repeated working through is necessary if the resident is to 'leave properly' (Wilson, 1985).

Nobody at Henderson seems quite sure what leaving properly means, although the phrase is liberally used and, sometimes, wielded as a stick with which to beat the resident into owning feelings of sadness. Leaving

properly certainly implies that some degree of planning, and agreement
with the community about the leaving itself, has taken place. In order to
facilitate this there is a 'leavers' small group, which takes place weekly
during small group time. Both practical and emotional issues are
explored and, optimally, resolved in this setting (Parker, 1989). Just as
the new residents have their own small group for the first three weeks,
which involves a senior resident, so the 'leavers' group involves a non-
leaving resident and this keeps the relevant information alive in the community's mind. Information from this group is regularly fed back into the
community meeting. Although there is currently no formal follow-up
treatment, prior to discharge many residents will set up supportive social
structures for themselves, sometimes incorporating further individual or
group psychotherapy.

Role of staff

The staff (approximately 25 whole-time equivalents) are multi-disciplin-
ary; uniforms are not worn and first names are used. There is a flattening
of the usual hierarchy of power and much blurring of conventional staff
roles, although individual staff do take responsibility for particular
aspects of community life. Importantly, continuity of staff among the
various therapy groups is maintained, as far as possible. Most staff
(nursing and social therapy) work on a rota, and others (medical, senior
nurse manager, social worker, art therapist and research psychologist)
work 9 a.m.–5 p.m., Monday to Friday. At night and at weekends there
are only two rota staff on duty, except for the Saturday morning community meeting, which is also attended by one of the medical staff. There
are no distinct night staff, and thus those on the rota cover both day and
night shifts, making continuity of staffing by rota staff sometimes problematic. But this also yields certain advantages, strengthening one fault
line along which the staff group may otherwise become 'split' or
polarised.

Staff meetings

There are daily multidisciplinary staff meetings, which take place at
morning handover and at lunchtime. Handover from day staff to night
staff, in the evening, also involves two of the residents. Staff meet after all
the main treatment groups to review and reflect on what has taken place.
There are also staff meetings that deal with business matters, mutual

supervision of clinical work (weekly), and a fortnightly academic meeting. The weekly staff sensitivity group is facilitated by an outside psychotherapist, and is set up to deal with staff–staff conflicts as they might relate to the professional context.

All staff meetings take place in group settings, and the flattened hierarchy means that decision-making, about the unit's business and internal management and clinical matters, is via negotiation and consensus. In this way staff are kept in touch with the reality of having to function as a group of more or less equals (despite obvious hierarchical aspects and differences). To an extent, this situation mirrors that of the residents, although the staff's working day is even more highly structured than theirs. Resultant time pressures on the staff, together with the group setting, potentially facilitate an empathic understanding of the residents' experience of being in the community, which is important since maintaining empathic contact with such a client group is not easy.

Themes

In many respects, staff experience and react to the community in the same way as do residents and the ideological themes outlined above, as identified by Rapoport, indicate the extent to which traditional staff roles are abandoned or blurred. In relation to the residents, the staff need to be facilitators rather than organisers or advisers. However, to succeed in this intention and provide the function of 'containment' is a difficult task, particularly in the face of aggressive or other antisocial or rule-breaking behaviour. In order to avoid simple retaliation to residents, it is important for staff to have some guiding philosophy and theoretical underpinning, and the various treatment processes and ideological themes already referred to offer some help. Other concepts that are used are transference and counter-transference and, in this respect, the abusing parent–child victim dynamic theme is prominently played out in various guises. Thus it may be that the staff group at any one time feels particularly abused, and condemning of the resident group. At other times, the staff group feels inordinately guilty that they have not been better providers or more ideal 'parent' figures (staff as abusers). Often, the dynamic is played out within the staff group itself where individual staff members or subgroups of staff are powerfully split or polarised into feeling as if they are victims or perpetrators in relation to other staff. The task is for staff to become aware of the pervasive influence of this and other dynamic and covert forces.

Parallel processes

There is an interesting phenomenon whereby at a given point in time issues to do with the residents, for example concerning the owning of responsibility, very closely mirror issues in the staff group. This phenomenon (isomorphism) can be made use of in terms of the staff dynamics illuminating those of the residents, and vice versa. Either set of dynamics can be explored with the aim of shedding light on the other. In this way, as far as is possible, a more distinct boundary can be drawn between what are rightly staff concerns and issues and what are those of the residents.

Working with a highly disordered client group, such as at Henderson, makes high demands on the professional capacity of staff members. To an extent the rigid structure of the system of staff meetings encourages a regression in staff to infantile modes of relating, with the possibility of abdicating responsibility for particular tasks because of blurring of staff roles. Even the flattening of the staff's hierarchical relationships does not necessarily facilitate mutual confrontation in relation to these important issues.

Leadership

The task of leadership in such a system of flattened hierarchy is a difficult balancing act with the temptation to become authoritarian and dictatorial often needing to be resisted, as far as possible, since its enactment may merely serve to reinforce dependency and irresponsibility in the rest of the staff team. These are the very aspects with which the resident group struggles and those which the staff group is paid to treat. Thus an important task for the leader is to facilitate staff–staff interaction at the same time as remaining an integral member of the team.

Conclusions

Other developments in psychiatric treatment since the inception of the therapeutic community, especially psychological and pharmacological therapies, have had the effect of restricting the successful application of the therapeutic community method. Thus the therapeutic community proper now has only limited application, for example, to patients suffering from psychotic illness, at least as the primary therapeutic intervention. Likewise, much of the treatment of mild, neurotic disorder has been taken over by other out-patient psychological treatments, whether cognitive-behavioural or psychodynamic. To some extent the therapeutic community territory represents that which has been unclaimed by other treatments, namely, many of those suffering from personality disorders, severe neuroses, eating disorders and the addictions, often found in combination in the same individual patient.

With the severely personality-disordered populations it is therapeutic community treatment that has been the most thoroughly researched and evaluated (Dolan and Coid, 1993). Even so, it is not always clearly predictable who within the personality-disordered client group can and who cannot benefit from therapeutic community treatment. This is because of a number of reasons, including difficulty with engagement in treatment and assessing true motivation for accepting treatment. Nevertheless, research demonstrates that a substantial number of personality-disordered patients can be helped by the therapeutic community method where other treatment has failed to produce lasting improvement (Whiteley, 1970; Copas *et al.*, 1983; Dolan *et al.*, 1992). Such success has been shown to be cost-effective, not least because of the relative cheapness of the non-drug group treatments involved. At 1992 prices, Henderson residents have been demonstrated to cost the UK's national resources approximately £14 500 in the year prior to admission. Their average stay, at 1992 prices, costs £23 000. Thus, given the demonstrated success rate of Henderson treatment in terms of lowered readmission to hospital and improved recidivism, the financial expenditure is justified. Short-term financial outlay by purchasing Health Authorities proved to be a sound investment (Menzies *et al.*, 1993).

References

American Psychiatric Association (1987) *Diagnostic and Statistical Manual of Mental Disorders.* 3rd edn. Washington: APA.

Clarke, D. (1965) The therapeutic community concept, practice and future. *British Journal of Psychiatry,* **111**, 947–54.

Copas, J. B., O'Brien, M., Roberts, J. C. and Whiteley, J. S. (1983) Treatment outcome in personality disorder: the effect of social, psychological and behavioural variables. *Personality and Individual Differences,* **5**, 565–73.

Derogatis, L. R., Lipman, R. S. and Covi, L. (1973) SCL-90: An outpatient psychiatric rating scale – preliminary report. *Psychopharmacology Bulletin,* **9**, 13–28.

Dolan, B. M. and Coid, J. (1993) *Psychopathic and anti-social personality disorders: treatment and research isues.* London: Gaskell.

Dolan, B. M., Evans, D. D. H. and Wilson, J. (1992) Therapeutic community treatment for personality disordered adults (1) Changes in neurotic symptomatology on follow-up. *International Journal of Social Psychiatry*, **38**(4), 243–50.

Dolan, B., Morton, A. and Wilson, J. (1990) Selection of admissions to a therapeutic community using a group setting: association with degree and type of psychological distress. *International Journal of Social Psychiatry*, **36**, 265–71.

Edelson, M. (1970) *Sociotherapy and Psychotherapy*. Chicago: University of Chicago Press.

Jones, M. (1952) *Social Psychiatry*. London: Tavistock Publications.

Jones, M. (1956) The concept of the Therapeutic Community. *American Journal of Psychiatry*, **112**, 647–50.

Jones, M. (1968) *Social Psychiatry in Practice*. Harmondsworth: Penguin.

Main, T. (1946) The hospital as a therapeutic institution. *Bulletin of the Menninger Clinic*, **10**, 66–8.

Main, T. (1983) The concept of the therapeutic community: variations and vicissitudes. In Pines, M. (ed.) *The evolution of group analysis*, pp. 197–217. London: Routledge and Kegan Paul.

Manning, N. (1989) *The Therapeutic Community Movement: Charisma and Routinisation*. London: Routledge.

Menzies, D., Dolan, B. and Norton, K. (1993) Funding treatment for personality disordered: Are short term savings worth long term costs? *Psychiatric Bulletin*, **17**, 517–19.

Norris, M. (1983) Changes in patients during treatment at Henderson Hospital therapeutic community during 1977–1981. *British Journal of Therapeutic Communities*, **1**, 147–58.

Norton, K. R. W. (1990) The significance and importance of the therapeutic community working practice. *International Journal of Therapeutic Communities*, **11**, 67–76.

Norton, K. R. W. (1992) A culture of enquiry – its preservation or loss. *International Journal of Therapeutic Communities*, **13**, 3–26.

Parker, M. (1989) Managing separation: the Henderson Hospital's 'Leavers' Group. *International Journal of Therapeutic Communities*, **10**, 5–15.

Rapoport, R. (1960) *The Community as Doctor*. London: Tavistock.

Whiteley, J. S. (1970) The response of psychopaths to a Therapeutic Community. *British Journal of Psychiatry*, **116**, 517–29.

Whiteley, J. S. (1986) Sociotherapy and psychotherapy in the treatment of personality disorder. Discussion paper. *Journal of the Royal Society of Medicine*, **79**, 721–5.

Wilson, J. (1985) Leaving home as a theme in a therapeutic community. *International Journal of Therapeutic Communities*, **6**, 71–8.

Part three
Postscript

16

A small group experience

JULIAN STERN

Introduction

A year before the conference I was approached by the organising committee, and invited to be a small group facilitator for four mornings at the conference from which this book derived. Although flattered by the invitation I was filled with trepidation. It seemed to me that any conference entitled 'Psychotherapy, Psychological Treatments and the Addictions' was at grave risk of becoming an idealistic attempt to span an unbridgeable gap between radically different fields of interest and areas of expertise. After all, don't many dynamic therapists refuse to work with people currently suffering from addictions? Don't most workers in the addictions field adopt a behaviourist approach with token economies and rewards and threats? How could one bridge the gaps? And how could one facilitate such a group?

In this brief and personal review, I will report back on what turned out to be a creative initiative – let's have groups first thing in the morning, with as wide a remit as desired. Let's talk about experiences as workers with addicts and alcoholics, as staff members in residential settings, as therapists, conference delegates, as humans with an interest in addicts and addiction. Let's talk, argue, listen, digest, think, feel.

I know there was anxiety in the small group members; what sort of a group is this, are we discussing patients and their problems, or our personal problems, or only problems raised by the conference? And I know there was anxiety in the facilitator – I felt unsure about how active to be, how transparent or opaque, how authoritarian or democratic, how interpretative or matter-of-fact. An out-patient detoxification clinic or an out-patient psychotherapy group felt much safer, and more familiar.

Psychodynamic therapists and analysts have written little about the addictions. Although many addicts may not be able to cope wth the rigours and relative deprivations implicit in psychoanalytic treatment, I

nonetheless believe that a psychodynamic approach can help explain
something about the addict's inner world, and something about his or
her relationship with carers, and the very strong responses evoked in the
carers. In preparing myself mentally for the conference and in particular
for the small groups, I took some inspiration from the work of the
British analyst Donald Winnicott (1967, published 1986). He was
addressing the Borstal Assistant Governor's Conference in
Winchester, and delivered a paper entitled 'Delinquency as a sign of
hope'. He explained ' . . . the second thing I want to make clear to you
is that I know I could not do your job. By temperament I am not fitted
for the work you do; and in any case I am not tall enough or big
enough. I have certain skills and a certain kind of experience, and it
remains to be seen whether there can be some pathway found between
the things that I know something about and the work that you are
doing. It might happen that nothing that I will say will have any effect
on what you do when you get back to your work. Nevertheless, there
might be some effect of an *indirect* kind, because it must sometimes
seem to you an insult to human nature that most of the boys and girls
you have to deal with have this tendency to be a nuisance'.

Here Winnicott explicitly recognised the different skills and aptitudes
needed for his job as a psychoanalyst, and theirs as Borstal governors. He
went on to link antisocial activity with deprivation, and then looked at
the ways in which a psychoanalytic approach might inform the work. He
made fewer claims for the value of psychoanalytic treatment, in particular arguing 'I think it may be impossible in most cases for those who are
in charge day and night to make the necessary adjustment in themselves
which would enable them to allow a boy a period of psychotherapy or
personal contact. What must be emphasised is the absolute difference
that there is in your attitude when you are responsible for general management, and when you are in personal relationship with the
child . . . For someone who is in charge, the antisocial activity is just
not acceptable. In the therapeutic session, by contrast, there is no question of morality except that which may turn up in the child.' Much of
what he wrote in 1967 seems equally pertinent to the position of a therapist working with people with addictions.

In trying to decide how best to report on the four morning groups, I
was faced with numerous dilemmas. A list of topics covered would be
tedious. An attempt at relating the precise content of each group would
be disrespectful of the confidentiality entrusted to me as facilitator, and
to each participant. So I shall restrict myself to some general comments

and themes, hopefully navigating a course between generalisations and detailed minutiae.

Splits, more splits, and healthy differences

In a group as diverse as ours, comprising psychiatrists, nurses, social workers, residential care workers, a psychologist, a GP and a psychotherapist, it is not surprising that splits emerged. At times they seemed like massive chasms. Is the addict by definition suffering from psychopathology or is he or she just a normal product of late twentieth century capitalism and inner city deprivation? Should the worker expose his or her own personality and personal life to the addict, or remain opaque? Is the person who walks into the clinic a patient, a client, a user, or an addict; a victim or an active agent and perpetrator? Should we as workers in the field socialise with 'them'?

As the days went on, the splits seemed less unbridgeable. Differences between group members were seen to be positive and even necessary. In the same ways as Winnicott acknowledged that he could not be a Borstal governor, yet was grateful that some people could, and chose to do so, so a healthy recognition of complementarity developed. In order to treat 'them', what is needed is a both/and approach – doctors and nurses, men and women, firm boundaries and empathic understanding. The unhealthy splits began to be transformed into healthy recognition of difference.

HIV and AIDS

On the afternoon preceding the third group, a panel discussion on HIV was held. The next day the group was dominated by HIV and AIDS. Extreme emotions were present. The horror of working with young adults confronting a terminal illness was vividly brought into the room, and it became clear how this issue can dominate all else. In a parallel manner, our attention was focused on the way in which policy makers too have focused on AIDS, and given new priority and funding to the addictions in the era of AIDS. Some workers expressed resentment at the way in which resources were channelled, others that not enough was being done for these tragic victims. Most contentious was the assertion that AIDS patients had in some way 'brought it upon themselves'. Once again a split emerged. Passive, tragic victims, or adults who have gambled with their own (and others') lives? How is it possible to retain a balanced viewpoint when working sometimes literally hands-on, with such a person? Is it possible (or desirable) to ignore one's own primitive fears about contamination, invasion by a virus, a virus sometimes sexually transmitted?

The discussion was heated and emotional. Life and death, morality and mortality evoke extreme passion. Both the passion and the reason are present in each one of us, the mix often critically affecting our choice of career, lifestyle, partner, or political affiliation. But as the week went on, once again, out of the divisions and splits a mutually respectful attitude seemed to emerge.

Addiction and perversion

The use of the word 'perversion' evokes strong feelings. Linked in most people's minds with judgementalism and sexual preference, it is a term also used by psychotherapists to refer to a particular relationship to truth, and to a pathological mode of coping with life's difficulties. It involves the denial of differences between generations, and between sexes. All of us, as the French analyst Chasseguet-Smirgel (1985) writes, have a perverse core, which is capable of being activated under certain circumstances. She writes 'All of us are open to the perverse solution which constitutes the balm for our wounded narcissism and a means of dissipating our feelings of smallness and inadequacy'. However, for some people, the perverse mode of functioning and thinking dominates, defence mechanisms such as splitting and disavowal, idealisation and denigration predominate. In such a schema, an addict uses perverse mechanisms to obliterate psychic reality and psychic pain. This view originates with Freud, who as early as 1905 distinguished the mental mechanisms in the neuroses from those of the perversions: 'Neuroses are, so to say, the negative of perversions'.

Much debate in the group centred on whether this is a useful way of looking at addicts and their 'psychic solution'. Once again, the group seemed polarised between some who saw such a viewpoint as pejorative, judgemental, unhelpful, conservative, and stigmatising, and others who felt it to be more useful.

The group process itself

There was, throughout the week, a tension as to the nature of the group. Was it to be didactic, therapeutic, personally exposing, academic, emotional? And what was the role of the facilitator – interpretative, clarifying, confrontational, observer or participant, therapist or colleague? The answer turned out to be all and none of the above.

As the week progressed, I detected a real sense of people coming together, a mutual appreciation of the work and thinking of the others in the group, a sense of a group of people committed to working with difficult patients, over long periods of time; of mutual respect, and of a recognition that the hands-on worker and the seemingly more remote academic require each other; that both possess and articulate areas which are often disowned in the other.

The cultural and professional diversity of the group members, from Asia, Africa and Europe, enriched proceedings; the commitment of participants to their work, their patients, and the pursuit of knowledge and understanding was obvious, and extended to punctual attendance of the groups at the unsociable hour of 8.30 a.m.!

On at least one feature there was agreement – that such work requires dedication and patience.

How poor are they that have not patience!
What wound did ever heal but by degrees?
Though know'st we work by wit, and not by witchcraft;
And wit depends on dilatory time.

Shakespeare: Othello, II, iii, 376

Following Chasseguet-Smirgel, I think the addict does reject 'dilatory time', this absence of witchcraft, and one conclusion unified all of us; that the 'quick fix' solutions of the addict cannot be mirrored in their carers.

Any report of such a group process is by definition a personal and biased viewpoint, but if the spirit of co-operation and mutual respect that was evident in the groups could continue, I believe our academic, professional and personal lives would be much enriched.

References and further reading

Bion, W. R. (1961) *Experiences in Groups*. London: Tavistock Publications

Chasseguet-Smirgel, J. (1985) *Creativity and Perversion*. London: Free Association Books.

Freud, S. (1905) Three essays on the theory of sexuality. In: Strachey, J. (ed.) *The Standard Edition of the Complete Psychological Works of Sigmund Freud*, Vol. 7, pp. 125–43. London: Hogarth Press.

Hinshelwood, R. (1987) *What Happens in Groups*. London: Free Associations Press.

Joseph, B. (1982) Addiction near to death. *International Journal of Psychoanalysis*, **63**, 449–56.

Winnicott, D. W. (1986) *Home is Where We Start From*. London: Penguin.

Index

hypnosis, 22

interventions, 84–8
see also brief therapy

Japan
amphetamines, 4
solvent abuse, 4

life cycle
age-specific developmental tasks,
31–3
dynamics, 37
individual and therapy, 33–6
life experiences, outcome of abuse, 12
Linehan, dialectical behaviour
therapy, 147–55
lone-parent families, 52–3

marijuana, and other drug use, 9
mental illness
impact on family, 49–51
parental, 50–1
methadone, 101–2, 167
Milan system, family therapy, 115–17
motivation, 162
ambivalence, 176–79
resolution, 180–2
attrition, 182–4
and natural recovery process, 229–5
in treatment of addictive behaviour,
173–88
motivational milieu therapy, 184
mutual help movements,
Washingtonians, 60–7
Alcoholics Anonymous, 220–39

neurosis, caused by substance
dependence, 97–100
neurosogenesis model, Freud, 21
Newcastle study, poverty, 48

onset of abuse, 5–6, 6–9

pattern, carry forward, 46–7
perversion, and addiction, 263
poverty, 48
precontemplation, 161, 190
see also stages of change
Prochaska, and DiClemente, stages of
change model, 161–2, 180,
189–205

Psychic Retreats, 88–91
psychotherapy
academic psychology, 19
aims, 30–8
case studies, 78–84
marital therapy, 78–9
clinical thinking, 19
defined, 98
interventions, 84–8
and life cycle, 19–43
nineteenth century, 58–73
psychoanalysis subject matter, 29
psychoanalytic models of mind and
symptom formation, 20–9
range of applicabilities, 38–9

relapse prevention, 163–4

schema-focused therapy, 139–6
self-invalidation, 149
single parents *see* lone-parent families
small groups, 260–4
smoking
cessation, 10–11
US fashion, 4
social cognition and motivational
issues, 174–6
social deviance, 6–9
see also conduct disorder
social disadvantage, 48–52
solution focused brief therapy, 123–37
solvent abuse, Japan, 4
stages of change, 161–2, 180, 189–205
definitions, 191–3
model, 190–1
movement throught the stage,
195–6
over two-year period, 201–2
process of change, 197
questionnaire, 198–201
scales (URICA), 193–5
stage-matched interventions, 203
states of change, 196–7
step families, 53–4
substance dependence, as neurosis,
97–100
substance misuse, behavioural
therapies, 158–71
suicide, 14
and parasuicide, 147, 153–4
symptom formation, and
management, 20–9